Critical Resilience for D0153441

The nursing profession is under pressure. Financial demands, student debt, the target culture, political scrutiny in the wake of major care scandals and increasing workloads are all taking their toll on professional morale and performance. This timely book considers the meaning of resilience in this adverse context and explains why measures to preserve individual nurses' and students' well-being are flawed if they don't take into account wider political and organizational perspectives.

Arguing that healthcare can be thought about and experienced differently, this book:

- provides a summary of the latest research on resilience, explaining its relevance and also limitations for nurses;
- considers debates about compassion and highlights the effects of policy agendas on nurse education and nursing work;
- re-evaluates nursing's professional identity, including where nursing has come from and the effects of class, gender and race on its powerbase;
- assesses the role of politics and social media, both in driving change and feeding resistance; and
- introduces the idea of critical resilience as a complete framework for resisting bullying and fostering survival and change in the nursing workforce.

Direct, upbeat, at times provocative and witty, this agenda-setting book enables nurses to understand why they feel the way they do. It also lists what opportunities are available to them to change, resist and survive in what has become a complex, challenging – if still deeply rewarding – line of work.

Michael Traynor is Professor of Nursing Policy at Middlesex University, London, UK, where he works in the Centre for Critical Research in Nursing and Midwifery.

Critical Resilience for Nurses

An Evidence-based Guide to Survival and Change in the Modern NHS

Michael Traynor

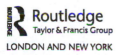

Routledge
Taylor & Francis Group

LONDON AND NEW YORK

First published 2017
by Routledge
2 Park Square, Milton Park, Abingdon, Oxon OX14 4RN

and by Routledge
711 Third Avenue, New York, NY 10017

Routledge is an imprint of the Taylor & Francis Group, an informa business

© 2017 M. Traynor

The right of Michael Traynor to be identified as author of this work has been asserted by him in accordance with sections 77 and 78 of the Copyright, Designs and Patents Act 1988.

British Library Cataloguing-in-Publication Data
A catalogue record for this book is available from the British Library

Library of Congress Cataloging in Publication Data
Names: Traynor, Michael, 1956– author.
Title: Critical resilience for nurses : an evidence-based guide to survival and change in the modern NHS / Michael Traynor.
Description: Abingdon, Oxon ; New York, NY : Routledge, 2017. | Includes bibliographical references.
Identifiers: LCCN 2016047469| ISBN 9781138194229 (hbk.) | ISBN 9781138194236 (pbk.) | ISBN 9781315638928 (ebk.)
Subjects: | MESH: Great Britain. National Health Service. | Nursing Process | Evidence-Based Nursing—methods | Resilience, Psychological | Empathy | Organizational Innovation | Burnout, Professional—prevention & control | Great Britain
Classification: LCC RT41 | NLM WY 100 FA1 | DDC 610.73—dc23
LC record available at https://lccn.loc.gov/2016047469

ISBN: 978-1-138-19422-9 (hbk)
ISBN: 978-1-138-19423-6 (pbk)
ISBN: 978-1-315-63892-8 (ebk)

Typeset in Sabon
by Florence Production, Stoodleigh, Devon, UK

Contents

Foreword

Written by the author's former colleague, filmmaker Jeremy Urquist.

I first met the author of this book while we were both training to be nurses at an institution I won't name. We met in the first week of the course and as we were somewhat older than the rest of the set we had a few things in common. At the end of what turned out to be a rather traumatic 3 years – more of that later – we went our separate ways. Instead of getting a job as a nurse, as most of our classmates did, for various reasons that I will not go into here, I developed a career for myself in documentary filmmaking. I had left the world of nursing far behind. Then something strange happened. While working in Buenos Aires in Argentina research-ing for a film about Jorge Luis Borges, quite out of the blue I bumped into Michael Traynor in a waiting room at the Hospital Británico. I had had a minor accident but I never found out what took Traynor to that rather impressive and reputedly efficient establishment. As we sat waiting we got to talking about the old days of our nurse training together and he reminded me about certain events that I had erased from my memory.

He told me about Miriam, who was one of our classmates, and the unfortunate events that befell her at the end of our training. As we sat there in the disinfected waiting room where a name was called out every 10 minutes or so and someone got up from their chair and shuffled off, we discussed at length whether when misfortune comes, it comes in some strange way at our own invitation.

Miriam had been an exemplary student and in fact had come from a family of nurses. Her mother and her grandmother, as well as her aunt, had all been in the profession. Miriam spoke of them with pride. I think that must have helped her to bear the difficult card she was dealt in her placements. On the very first day of her first ward a patient had died while Miriam was helping her to wash. I remember Miriam telling us afterwards that she had been getting irritated with the patient because she seemed to be refusing to help herself. On her second placement she was accused of trying to steal controlled drugs from the ward. Then, while out on community experience, the car being driven by her mentor was involved in an accident and as a result her mentor, an experienced community nurse, spent months in hospital and in fact never worked as a nurse again. Miriam seemed to take all this adversity in her stride. During the second year of training Miriam's mother died of cancer. The readiness with which Miriam returned to work after this challenging event surprised and impressed us at the time. Her final year of training, mercifully, went without incident so it was all the more surprising to hear that shortly after qualifying she had one day disappeared from the ward she was working on and it was later discovered that she had taken her own life.

Eventually my name was called out and our conversation was interrupted. When I returned from my minor treatment, carrying a small paper bag of painkillers, Traynor had gone. I was surprised but being under pressure to meet one of Borges' relatives who had agreed to talk to me, I left the hospital and did not give this chance meeting much thought.

Nearly 2 years later, Traynor contacted me out of the blue and told me about a project that he was working on and asked if I would be interested in writing a foreword for this book. That the topic was resilience did not surprise me, given our conversation in Argentina. His intention was that I write something from the perspective of a maker of documentaries, true stories about real people, but I have chosen instead to relate this brief conversation I had with the author because I believe that it gives some explanation for Traynor's personal interest in the topic, as well as its importance. I have the feeling that Miriam's story has hovered over him like a spectre.

Author's introduction

A spectre is haunting nursing. What is this spectre if not an unspoken anxiety? This anxiety emerges in a hospital or clinic when as a student nurse you are placed in positions of trust and authority but know you lack the knowledge you need to take up that position with confidence. Either you learn to survive this, or you leave. And rates of drop out from nursing courses in the UK are 'as high as 30 per cent' (Lintern 2013). But this loss has a flipside. In the face of pressures to cut the corners of care, to get more done with fewer staff and sicker patients some of those that stay in the profession, often for many years, fail to stand up for nursing values. Recent scandals have shone the media spotlight on this problem often described as the loss of values and morale. Nursing 'failures' are seen by some as caused by the weight of sustained adversity (Francis 2013b).

These are some of the difficult problems that organizations and those within them are charged with tackling – dropout and burnout. So it is easy to see the attraction of one single solution. I claim in this book that resilience has been proposed and taken up as just such a solution. It bypasses the proliferation of problems, each with their own intricate set of causes, and aims directly at the spectre of anxiety. But this solution puts the onus entirely on the character of the individual nurse. My argument is that the promotion of resilience comes at a price and that for survival and change you need a different kind of tactic entirely.

I start this book by describing the origins of the idea of resilience in child psychology and psychiatry as well as definitions, debates, differences and developments within the field. Chapter 1 should give you a working knowledge of the concept. In Chapter 2, I go on to summarize critiques of the recent focus on resilience. My own critique of 'traditional' resilience is twofold: first the way the notion has been taken up is problematic, and second the concept itself seems to exhibit some circularity, by which I mean that explanations of the mysterious inner quality of resilience seem to often be based on other mysterious inner qualities. Though later and more sophisticated research points to ecological i.e. environment-based contributions to resilience, I argue that the popular promotion, as well as its uptake in nursing, features a strong focus on resilience as an individual capacity that people can make efforts to develop.[1] I then introduce an alternative that I call critical resilience. These first two chapters, then, provide you with a summary of ideas about resilience and some of their problems. In a few sentences that are crucial to the whole book I will point out the difference between complaint and critique. The critically resilient nurse does not spend the day complaining, but spends it developing exciting critiques. The rest of the book presents material that lays the foundation for your own critical resilience.

First, there are three chapters about nursing work. In the first of these I look at the idea of compassion, much talked about today. Without straying into the content of these chapters, I want to alert you to the fact that you will find the phrase 'the idea of . . .' or 'talk of . . .' scattered throughout this book prefixing key terms such as compassion and resilience itself. I want to say before we go further that a crucial part of being critical is, I think, being sceptical about terminology, particularly if it is often used. In fact, as I have written this book I have been surprised when I have looked into concepts like resilience or empathy, another term often used in nursing, to find the problem not so much in the concepts themselves, although the way they are generated always reflects their context, but with the way they

---

1 It is as if 'resilience' has become a separate colloquial term, bearing only a passing resemblance to the original concept developed by psychologists.

have been taken up by particular groups and used to promote certain interests and projects. Chapter 3 adopts this approach to ask where today's emphasis on care and compassion in nursing came from and to investigate the uses and abuses of the terms. Chapter 4 presents a body of evidence that has shown nursing and healthcare work as stressful (as if you didn't know). This includes psychological studies of burnout, the idea of emotional labour, as well as ethnographies describing the subtle and often creative and informal ways that clinicians interact with organizations to get the work done, to manage their own potential trauma and for other reasons. Chapter 5 delves into history to account for nursing's identity: for example, it is unusual today for an occupation to be so identified with one particular gender. If it is true that most human societies are patriarchal, i.e. men and the power of men tend to shape how that society is run and who is rewarded, then nursing has had to develop ways of resisting. I will talk about some responses to this predicament, one being complaint on the part of many nurses. I will describe some more productive approaches.

Political systems and politicians are the subject of Chapter 6. I will argue that for the most part politicians are uninterested in nursing and that often the only government policy to affect nursing is policy aimed at solving some other problem such as the rising cost of medicine, healthcare scandals or the number of migrants entering the UK. Understanding politics can help you understand the daily work of nursing. Chapter 7 focuses on the actual context that the majority of nurses in the UK work in – NHS hospitals, clinics and other services. A large amount of the difficulty that nurses and doctors experience in their day-to-day work arises from the organization of their work – they are like members of medieval guilds trying to work in modern bureaucracies. Added to that, if you are a student nurse you face another kind of split between the service itself and the university system where you are taught how to nurse. It is to university tutors, for example, that you might reveal that you have witnessed poor care or been the victim of bullying or racism. This chapter talks about this possible tension and suggests creative ways through. I give advice on how to handle bullying.

Being critical in the sense that it is used in this book emerges from a particular theoretical orientation. Chapter 8 sets out that orientation and the theories associated with it. I argue that compared with what might be called common sense, theory can make the world look a very different place. Critical theory can be empowering and liberating because it gives you a framework which can help you make sense of life's complex array of people, organizations and experiences. After a while, thinking theoretically becomes a practice – it is how you are in the world, resilient because you are informed and no longer naïve.

The topic of the last chapter, Chapter 9, is nursing solidarity, organizing and resistance and the focus is on how social media can help. Sometimes it seems that professional organizations and employers see the social media phenomenon predominantly either as a source of anxiety or an opportunity for rather uninspiring self-promotion. This chapter argues that social media provide important and stimulating network-building and organizing opportunities that are non-geographical and asynchronous, particularly valuable perhaps for the individual whose views make them isolated among their colleagues. #BursaryOrBust is a good example of a Twitter hashtag adopted by student activists who used social media to share information about the government's plan to replace the student nurse bursary with an interest-accruing loan, to organize protests and to make links with other radical groups.

Now a word about who this book is for. This book was originally aimed specifically at nursing students because my research had suggested that they (you – if you are such a student) were most in need of the support that a sophisticated and intelligent understanding of nursing work could give. It is clear to me that as a group student nurses have little power in the nursing and NHS hierarchies and at times feel the most vulnerable. While the 'problem' of attrition may not be as serious as some make out there is little doubt that many are unprepared for the shock that starting nursing work involves. What is more, many students that stick the course – and the vast majority of course do – experience stress and unhappiness that to some extent could be eased with this same confident and critical understanding. For these reasons I originally wrote the book for this group. However, it was suggested to me that those nurses who are already qualified may also be in need of a book that supports them at times of pressure with a discussion of some of the causes of problems – and pressure – in healthcare and nursing. Finally it was suggested that university lecturers in nursing may also find the discussion that this book starts a useful resource for their scholarly and teaching work with students. So I have written for a wider range of readers than originally intended. Some parts of the book may be more relevant to some groups than others though it will all be of interest and entertainment to every reader.

The idea for the 'evidence-based' part of the book's title also came at the suggestion of reviewers of my original proposal to the publisher. Since the term 'evidence-based medicine' and other 'evidence-based' variants first took off in the UK as adjectives applied to healthcare 15 years ago, the term still has currency as a marker of seriousness and reliability. I included it in the title here to signal that the debates that form the majority of this book are debates about research findings and their implications and that I include material from my own research throughout. However, despite the association in many people's minds of science with objectivity, research is an unavoidably social and political activity, for example in terms of what gets on the agenda for research funding and what does not. I do not believe that it would be possible, and certainly not interesting, to produce an 'objective' book about resilience. My sense is that some resilience researchers are strongly committed to social justice and advocate for social policy aimed at promoting this based on the findings of good quality research. I cannot resist the suspicion, however, that other researchers (or the same researchers at different moments) are far more orientated around the technical challenges of measurement and just do not approach understanding the political context in which resilience might be promoted with the same degree of attention or understanding. My challenge in this book is to put this kind of research as it has been applied to nursing work into this new context, pointing to some of the cultural and political influences on the research process. And that challenge is part of a political and research tradition that has gone under the name of 'critical' as Chapter 8 sets out. One critical writer says that 'the idea of freedom as a purely interior reality which is always there even when men are enslaved is typical of the idealist [i.e. non-critical] mentality' (Horkheimer 1972 p. 230). Some expressions of resilience seem close to claiming just this.

Survival and change: these are the outcomes that this book is imagining for you the reader, possibly in that order. Classic resilience research investigated those who appeared to survive adverse events and circumstances. As I have just said, having a sophisticated framework to interpret and make sense of events and circumstances can also aid survival but I am highly sceptical about 'survival' as an end point in itself. It is too easy for managers or educators to see survival as an answer to their problems – at least partly because they are penalized for staff turnover or student attrition: 'teach students some "resilience" and they may last that bit longer before finally succumbing to disillusionment and by then it will be somebody else's problem.' I do not know whether this is naivety, cynicism or panic on their part – or a genuine desire to do the best thing when options are limited. It is probably all of them. The causes of the adversity that might lead to the need for resilience in the first place are silently acknowledged as too difficult to deal with and so nothing changes, or rather when it does, we have not been part of the discussion. It is also possible in some circumstances that 'survival' may be part of the problem rather than part of the solution. In some circumstances it may be better politically and personally to leave than to 'survive'. The Radical Nursing Group from the 1980s made badges that read 'I refuse to cope', referring to the widespread sense that nurses will continue to work in increasingly constrained and dysfunctional environments.

Critical resilience has a built-in concern for change. 'Philosophers have hitherto only *interpreted* the world in various ways; the point is to *change* it' (Marx 1845). What might change mean? In the healthcare context it can take many shapes. Formally the NHS wants to encourage 'change agents', those individuals who are not numbed by traditional ways of working and who have the imagination and charisma to inspire teams or whole organizations to work differently perhaps to address a problem with patient throughput or safety issues. This is one kind of change. Reading this book may give you enough of an understanding of organizations to enable you to participate in or instigate this kind of activity. It can be of huge value and improve patient experience and even save lives. Those nurses I admire are involved in a different kind of change that originates from a fundamental critique of the profession's contradictions, limited realm of power and self-knowledge. One of these has become a policy activist on an international stage although she started out as a campaigner and troublemaker at a local level. Another is a more invisible figure but her long-standing and critical blog has found its way into the bookmarks and, I believe, the consciousness of a growing number of nurses and other NHS figures. I discuss this further in Chapter 9. Speaking truth to power, as both of these individuals do, is part of changing the status quo simply by changing the way a topic is talked about publicly. Critical resilience can be understood as resistance. Perhaps this word should have been in the book's title too.

Throughout the book I have included special material: invitations for you to engage in thought experiments, often to imagine how present arrangements could be different. These appear in shaded boxes. I have also started chapters with quotations from student nurses speaking in focus groups that I have been running for the last 5 years. Sometimes their relevance is obvious. Sometimes it is more to plant the seed of an idea or an emotion that might develop in parallel to your reading of the material of the chapter. Naturally I have used pseudonyms in these quotations – apart from my own interventions because anonymity makes me nervous. Then there are the footnotes. In many books these are used for more detailed material. Because I want this book to be readable, I use them to provide expansion, explanation or slight diversions that some readers may want to follow. However, I also see footnotes as comedy opportunities.

If you want to contact me about anything you have read in this book, you are very welcome. I have created a web page for responses and discussion at *michael-traynor.net*.

My email address is m.traynor@mdx.ac.uk

Acknowledgements

As ever, I would like to thank my collaborators at the Centre for Critical Research in Nursing and Midwifery for their companionship and support. I also thank all my colleagues at Middlesex University for being such stimulating and convivial people to work with. I thank Jane Salvage whose intellectual support and example I greatly value. Great appreciation also to Hephzibah Rendle-Short who edited the first two paragraphs of this book.

Jeremy Urquist acknowledges the influence of The Atlas Group Archive (www.theatlasgroup.org/index.html) in shaping approaches to documentary work.

Chapter 1

Resilience: where did it come from?

Research on resilience and its use in nursing

MICHAEL: Can you tell me the difference between a good clinical placement and a bad one?

PENNY (third-year Adult branch student): I'd say good is how the ward is run, so if it's an organized ward, they know you're coming; they know how to look after a student -

MICHAEL: Which is how?

PENNY: Making you feel welcome, supporting and teaching you, cause obviously we do placement for free, pretty much, if, like I've always said, if I go to a placement and they teach me, I'm not bothered that I'm not getting paid, because it's a learning opportunity. But if I'm going somewhere and your mentor's not even interested in you, none of the staff, they see a student as a burden, that is what makes a bad placement, for me anyway . . .

DAVE: Yeah, maybe it's not about personality but it's about that they are overwhelmed with work, so they are very nice people and very helpful, but, because they are overwhelmed by work and they are very stressed, they just don't really bother about having us students, because they have six other patients to look after, so they don't have time to look after the student.

In this chapter I set out some definitions of resilience. But definitions are of little help if you want to understand an idea. It is more useful to know where that idea came from or, in other words, how it got here. So I start by summarizing the origins of the concept and its development from studies of particular population groups through to investigations of resilience among nurses.

Origins of research into resilience: psychoanalysis and trauma

Few would argue today with the idea that childhood events have a lasting impact throughout adult life. But before Freud's psychoanalytic theories[1] developed at the turn of the nineteenth and twentieth centuries such ideas would have been uncommon or at least not considered a subject worthy of scientific investigation. Because of Freud's position – as a doctor attempting to treat patients with sometimes incapacitating problems – his focus was on psychopathology, literally the study of the suffering of the soul. Often suffering was related, he found, to traumatic events in childhood. His first patient who has come to be known as 'Anna O' found that talking about her symptoms freely and retrieving memories of traumatic incidents she had experienced led to some relief of those symptoms. From this practice Freud developed his 'talking cure' and an elaborate range of theories that he refined throughout his life. Fundamental to them is the notion of the unconscious, the continual repression of thoughts that are too difficult or traumatic to process consciously of which the individual is unaware yet which influence thought, emotion and behaviour. Freud was interested in the effects of trauma on the individual and their expression in talk and behaviour, sometimes in bizarre symptoms. Though based in extended and painstaking clinical work, his theories in many ways run counter to prevailing ideas and common sense. His work remains controversial.

The work of Freud and his colleagues provided a fertile ground for later psychological studies of childhood but the field became characterized by strong divisions and rival theories and approaches. Attachment theory developed by John Bowlby (1907–1990) emerged from and challenged Freud's theories. Bowlby, whose own childhood was characterized by distant and interrupted relationships with his parents, focussed his work on the child's early environmental experiences and found that

---

1   Sigmund Freud (1856–1939), an Austrian doctor and neurologist, considered the 'father' of psychoanalysis.

separation from a primary care giver was often associated with trauma at the time and sometimes social and emotional problems in later life. Bowlby's ideas, first presented in the late 1950s and early 1960s, caused anxiety among the followers of Freud. The key difference between them was that Bowlby's focus was on observable events in the child's upbringing while Freud and his followers believed that it was the events that occurred in the imagination of the child that provided the source of psychic problems. From the Freudian point of view, there is no way of telling from observing behaviour alone the meaning of that behaviour for the individual. We will return to this line of argument in Chapter 2. A second difference concerned focus. Bowlby developed a theory of child development that he claimed had the advantage that it was built on observation of the normal child rather than extrapolated from clinical work with already damaged individuals (Gullestad 2001). There are very many accounts of the origins of 'resilience' research and it is rare to find Bowlby mentioned in these but his theory of the benefits of attachment and his interest in the effects of childhood trauma coupled with his concern for direct observation of environmental events impinging on the child set the context for later studies.[2] Succeeding researchers have considered the presence of at least one healthy attachment to a significant adult as a precondition of resilience in children (Earvolino-Ramirez 2007).

James Anthony (1916–2014), one of the first child psychiatrists to write at length about the topic of resilience and vulnerability, collaborated with Bowlby as well as Anna Freud (daughter of Sigmund Freud) in his early career. Anthony saw the origins, or rather the forerunners, of research on human resilience in two areas. One, perhaps surprisingly, lay in laboratory experiments in which rats were placed in various types of extreme environments and observed to respond in very different ways,

2   Michael Rutter, a resilience researcher, considered that Bowlby overestimated the damage caused by infantile separation Rutter, M. (1985). "Resilience in the face of adversity: Protective factors and resistence to psychiatric disorder." *British Journal of Psychiatry* **147**: 598–611.

some 'seemingly thrived on it' (Anthony and Cohler 1987, p. 4). The second was epidemiological studies that had showed varied susceptibility to coronary heart disease in particular populations as well as the apparent capacity of some individuals to live through major social and other life changes 'and yet exhibit little if any overt evidence of illness' (p. 5). Anthony and others focussed on child development in conditions of social disadvantage and were fascinated by the same apparent ability of some children to survive disadvantage. They used the term 'invulnerable' in a possibly awkward attempt to label this phenomenon. Anthony himself drew some similarities between these 'invulnerables' and the detached and sociopathic character Meursault from Albert Camus' 1942 novel *L'Etranger* (The Outsider). When Meursault's mother dies, for example, he is mildly irritated rather than deeply affected. This gives an indication of Anthony's nuanced approach to the notion of resilience. Anthony drew on Freud's ideas of the psyche's defensive structures that protect against the impact of strong external stimuli in his explorations of the individual's response to its environment. However, for him, the most efficient protective system took the form of the infant's caregiver and her (for many researchers the caregiver was generally the mother) actions and precautions.

In the years after Freud, some psychoanalysts chose to focus more on the role of the ego than on the unconscious forces at work in the individual, trying to shift the field away from psychopathology onto more positive ground. So it is not surprising that research into resilience came to emphasize the 'coping' work that the ego was considered to engage in (known as 'ego-resilience') rather than unconscious defences, although some claimed that the two worked in harmony together (Moriarty and Toussieng 1976). In addition, effective personal coping could take place in environments that were more or less encouraging of self-reliance and researchers also commented that there was 'nothing out of the ordinary' in such resilience-enabling situations. From observation, researchers began to develop inventories of the apparent characteristic behaviour of 'good copers' along with questionnaires designed to assess the presence of these factors e.g. (Murphy and Moriarty 1976).[3] So to summarize this part of its history, early research on resilience paints a picture of internal and environmental factors that interact and change during developmental periods of children.

A debate develops: can resilience be grown?

One of the continuing debates among resilience researchers has concerned two related questions 'Is resilience essentially a personal characteristic – a character trait – or a dynamic developmental process?' (Earvolino-Ramirez 2007 p. 76). The second question flows from this: 'and if it is a developmental process, can it be taught or improved by external intervention?' I will talk more about how the second question played out later in this chapter. The more dynamic idea of resilience necessarily involves two components. The first is the adversity to which the individual responds. The second is the response, 'rebounding' or 'reintegrating' by returning to 'normal life', or 'coping'. Some writers also add that the response involves a positive personal growth, similar to the popular idea that some types of people 'thrive on adversity'.

Researchers focussed their work on identifying sources of vulnerability on the one hand and on the other protective factors that could modify the harmful impact of adverse circumstances. It is important to remember that the flavour of this research is largely a result of its focus on children and young people growing up in some kind of disadvantaged background. In this context, vulnerability might include having parents with a mental health problem, living in a poor urban neighbourhood or low intelligence. Researchers began to produce lists of 'protective factors or processes' though some were at pains to point out protective factors are contextual, situational and individual and lead to varying outcomes (Johnson and Wiechelt 2004). For example, both vulnerabilities and protective factors can be

---

3   Its use is said to require 'hair-splitting judgements that can only be acquired through prolonged use' (Anthony and Cohler 1987 p. 19).

perating at the community, family or individual level (Luthar and Cicchetti 2000). At each of these levels supportive relationships with adults in school, emotionally responsive family caregiving and an easy-going temperament could be considered protective. Nevertheless despite the complicated way that these protective factors might interact with other elements of context, researchers devised questionnaires aimed at measuring the presence of such factors. For example, the Resilience Scale for Adults is a questionnaire with 37 questions designed to assess what the authors believe are the five dimensions of resilience: personal competence, social competence, family coherence, social support and personal structure (Friborg *et al.* 2003). The scale was devised based largely on the lists of protective factors developed by some of the preeminent resilience researchers over the previous 20 years and was created specifically to measure the presence of these attributes (Friborg *et al.* 2003). Other researchers have produced summaries of the protective factors labelled by six of the major resilience researchers. One lists 28 personal characteristics or skills, for example 'good natured, easy temperament' and 'decision-making ability' (Earvolino-Ramirez 2007). The single factor that relates to the individual's context, 'informal social support network', is assessed by asking the individual to rate it so there is an almost total focus on the individual.

Even though it could be said that by 2000, the 'dynamic' view of resilience had won the day, in the years leading up to this some researchers downplayed the contribution of social and environmental factors to resilience on the grounds that it is difficult to distinguish between the positive and negative effect of the same kind of social relationships (a marriage can be supportive but a divorce is likely to be threatening) and focus on internal protective factors instead (Rutter 1985). Perhaps these investigators felt that their skills and training equipped them better to investigate and measure the so-called internal world of individuals – anxiety, personality, IQ, etc. – rather than the messy and uncontrollable world of social relations and environmental contexts.

Some researchers have been at pains to point out dangerous misconceptions and simplifications of the idea of resilience that may arise as it is communicated from scientists to the public and to policymakers. The key, they emphasize, is the argument that resilience is not a personal characteristic of the individual but a term that might be applied to developmental trajectories, or in other words:

> many characteristics that appear to reside in the child are in fact continually shaped by interactions between the child and aspects of his or her environment.
>
> (Luthar and Cicchetti 2000 p. 864)

They explicitly raise the danger of policymakers falling back on common sense ideas of resilience as a kind of 'exceptional sturdiness' and of politicians misunderstanding or misusing the ideas raised by resilience research to blame vulnerable individuals for not possessing this ability and therefore reducing social support to these groups (Luthar and Cicchetti 2000 p. 864).

Not all researchers have been as clear-minded about these potential hazards. Consider these two statements by researchers about the importance of resilience research relative to broader social programmes:

> Some sources of adversity are preventable such as child maltreatment and it is far more effective to try to prevent these in the first place.
>
> (Masten and Obradovic 2006)

> The primary concern of those working with children and adolescents at risk is the prevention of maltreatment and abuse, but given that this is not always possible, the promotion of resilience is even more valuable.
>
> (Williams and Hazell 2011 cited in Winders 2014 p. 7)

The humanistic attraction of the study of the children who rise from adversity is summed up well by James Anthony at the close of the introduction to his book *The Invulnerable Child*. He starts by quoting contemporary resilience research and then goes on to offer his own conclusion:

> with our nations torn by strife between races and between social classes, these 'invulnerable' children remain the 'keepers of the dream' . . . Were we to study the forces that move such children to survival and adaptation, the long range benefits to our society may be far more significant than our many efforts to construct models of primary prevention designed to curtail the incidence of vulnerability.
>
> (Anthony and Cohler 1987 p. 46)

Four waves of resilience research?

Resilience research has changed since its early days. Some involved in the field have proposed that there have been 'four waves' of research, each building on the last with researchers becoming more aware of the ecological context in which adversity develops and the individual responds (Masten 2007). Whether we agree with this analysis or not, resilience has certainly been turned to by researchers across vastly different subject areas – from efforts to build in resilience to military systems, to town planning and marine ecology. The Stockholm Resilience Centre has produced a definition of the term that is a long way from the checklists of personality characteristics and skills that we have been looking at up to now. That organization sees resilience as 'the capacity [of a system] to use shocks and disturbances like a financial crisis or climate change to spur renewal and innovative thinking' (Stockholm Resilience Centre 2012 p. 3).[4] With this broadening out of the concept of resilience

---

4   As I have been writing this chapter, news has come in of terrorist attacks in Paris in which 130 people have been killed as they went about their Friday evening activities. I am wondering how that city will respond.

as our background we can now turn to look at resilience and nursing. An Internet search for these two terms turns up articles on how nurses can aid the resilience of particular patient groups (e.g. Molina *et al.* 2014) but it is on work on nurses' own resilience that I want to focus.

Resilience and nursing

There are two types of writing on resilience in nursing: editorials along with articles discussing the need for resilience among nurses on the one hand and on the other various research studies that set out to measure resilience, compare it with other characteristics of nurses or improve it through various interventions. Most of this research is done by nurses though some is carried out by psychologists and some is by nurses working for psychology-based qualifications. I will summarize the second type of writing – the research work – because it is more substantial and is where we would expect to find the most rigorous and cutting edge work on the topic. I looked at 15 varied articles that have appeared in leading nursing research journals over the last 10 years. See the Appendix for more details of these papers.

Research on resilience among nurses tends to have certain common features:

1   The authors start by listing contemporary features of nursing work that make it highly stressful and therefore comparable to the 'adversity' that classic resilience studies deal with to argue that resilience is highly applicable to nurses. These stressful factors have two origins: those that are intrinsic to the work itself and those that are a result of contemporary demographic, economic and political forces. The first group

If it re-emerges with renewed solidarity, calm and strengthened integration of marginalized migrant sectors of its society we could perhaps say that the Parisians have shown their city to be resilient against attacks of this kind.

of sources of stress include exposure to patient suffering and death and the close relationships that may develop with these patients (e.g. Zander *et al.* 2010, Dolan *et al.* 2012). The second group, which is referred to more often and at greater length, includes global nursing shortages and high turnover (e.g. Larrabee *et al.* 2010 p. 82), political change and under-resourcing of public healthcare (Koen *et al.* 2011), casualization, staff shortages, bullying, abuse and violence (e.g. Jackson *et al.* 2007).

The authors argue that continued stress and pressure and the possibility of burnout has effects on absenteeism, intention to leave, psychological morbidity and poor patient care. Some authors set out the economic cost of staff turnover in nursing at great length.[5] There is a broad assumption across this writing that for a nurse to remain in the nursing workforce is a free choice that can point to a degree of resilience and that some of those who remain apparently 'thrive' on the adversity they experience. There is also an assumption that a decision to leave nursing can be understood as succumbing to adversity, i.e. a negative consequence, a sign of pathology.[6] The articles tend to note that there is apparently unexplained variation between staff in similar roles who 'remain well' while others experience psychological distress.

2   Much research focuses on nursing specialities claiming them to be especially difficult to work in and so particularly in need of a resilient workforce (and of resilience research); for example aged care, intensive care, mental health, palliative care, renal nursing and paediatric oncology. I read

---

5   For example, 'Turnover cost per nurse ranged from $62,000 to $67,000 in a recent study (Jones, 2005), and results of another study (Waldman *et al.* 2004) indicated that the annual nurse turnover cost for an academic medical centre ranged from 3.4% to 5.8% of the organization's budget.'

6   None of the work I read mentions the possibility that nurses might remain in nursing because of lack of alternatives nor that leaving the profession could be seen as a sign of strength and appropriate 'adaptation' to use a psychological term often associated with resilience.

these claims as justification for research in these areas and suggest that any type of nursing work can be extremely difficult for any of the reasons mentioned above.

3   There is a tendency to take understandings and definitions (often brief) of resilience either entirely (Cameron and Brownie 2010) from other nursing literature or to rely heavily on it (Matos *et al.* 2010) so that key debates and nuances in the field are ignored and subsequent authors who rely heavily on nursing literature seem unaware of them.[7] The nursing literature tends to draw on an 'internal' understanding of resilience as 'a positive personality characteristic' (Matos *et al.* 2010 p. 309).

4   Following on from the above, while 'adversity' is understood in organizational and workforce terms there is little attempt to measure this with a focus that is almost entirely on individual personal response and characteristics. Most studies are carried out in single sites so there is no opportunity to investigate whether any differences in resilience are associated with different ways of working (rather than differences in individuals). The one author who compared resilience scores across two sectors, the for-profit and the highly stretched public sector in South Africa, found apparently higher resilience among private sector nurses (Koen *et al.* 2011) suggesting paradoxically that less adversity is associated with apparently higher resilience.

5   The studies that describe initiatives aimed at fostering resilience among nurses are individual-based. This focus on the individual is very different from the community-based programmes described in the child psychology literature. There is no conception or consideration of resilient systems in the nursing literature. Also comparisons are made with

---

7   For example some early models of resilience picture resilience as a personality trait that is stable over time however, contemporary perspectives of resilience emphasize a transactional-ecological model of human development where the individual is constantly interacting with the environment and adapting to its demands.

resilience studies of people with chronic or life-threatening disease though there is a fundamental difference in that members of an occupation are, in principle at least, able to walk away from their work-based adversity or move into positions of influence to change it. The evidence from resilience research suggests that it is important that those planning interventions recognize the mutual interactions between the individual and different aspects of their environments, as attempts to improve particular protective factors are likely to be ineffective on their own (Luthar and Cicchetti 2007 cited in Winders 2014).

6   There is circularity in some of the research where researchers ask nurses to talk about themselves in relation to resilience. For example, one group of authors (Cameron and Brownie 2010) tell us 'Nurses were encouraged to reflect on the following statement: "Resilience is the ability to rebound from adversity and overcome difficult circumstances in one's life".' As a response participants appear to identify factors that promote job satisfaction but label these 'in their own words' as resilience. This supports the researchers' belief in the importance of the operation of resilience.

7   Finally there is a tacit acknowledgement and a sense of powerlessness from the authors that the workplace experienced by nurses is so dysfunctional that it is better to invest energy in devising personal approaches to coping than investigating or challenging the causes of dysfunction. This is on the basis that 'nurses' occupational settings will always contain elements of stressful, traumatic or difficult situations, and episodes of hardship' (Jackson *et al.* 2007 p. 7), or 'it is important to acknowledge that work stress and crises are inevitable and even necessary for the growth and maturity of the individual and to allow them to reach their full potential' (Manzano García and Carlos 2012 p. 105). Another author considers that understanding resilience among nurses 'would provide hospital managers with useful guidelines for in-service training that won't be threatening and can facilitate growth in professional nurses' (Koen *et al.* 2011 p. 3). Promoting resilience among

nurses is a way, according to many of the authors, of reducing turnover in the nursing workforce, with the promise that 'nurses can thrive at the bedside for "extended periods of time" (Mealer *et al.* 2012 p. 297). Measuring resilience can also be used to identify those nurses with low resilience and target them for 'support' to help them to last longer. It is hard to resist the suspicion that this approach, with the intention of protecting nurses, promotes the status quo by trying to avoid a crisis in healthcare systems that might actually bring about some policy action.

Clearly resilience researchers in nursing are responding to the all too real difficulties experienced by nurses in the workplace. Faced with the complexity and power of the forces that determine the shape of healthcare worldwide – government policy, powerful other professions, large corporations – they take the understandable approach of exploring strategies for personal survival, or rather a particular limited range of these. I will save my critique of the unintended consequences of this approach for the next chapter although I have mentioned some of these in my summary of the research above.

I want to finish this chapter by summarizing what we know about resilience and resilience research:

- The idea emerged from the study of children who experienced 'adversity' during their upbringing and often this adversity was caused by, or featured social disadvantage
- The enigma was that children appeared to develop in very different ways given an apparently similar range of adversities
- Researchers have emphasized the crucial interaction between the child and their environment which can be relatively encouraging of resilience or discouraging
- Despite this knowledge of interaction many researchers have focussed their efforts on a search for personal qualities or skills that might be associated with greater resilience and some have attempted to intervene in ways designed to raise levels of resilience

- Resilience has also been seen as a key for other more complex situations and systems
- Research on resilience among nurses has tended to reflect the individual emphasis within the field rather than the ecological.

Chapter 2

The limits of resilience: introducing 'critical resilience'

YASMIN (third-year Adult branch student nurse): I also can't watch hospital programmes without being critical [laughs]. Like, if you watch Grey's Anatomy and stuff like that, that so wouldn't happen [laughs].

REEM: Telly CPR makes me cringe.

YASMIN: Yeah, they're all like, make-up in place, hair in place –

REEM: Bendy arms!

YASMIN: No, you would be sweating!

In this chapter I summarize the attractions of resilience but also its limitations and dangers; I suggest that an idea like resilience comes to prominence for many reasons; I set out an alternative to resilience that I am calling critical resilience; I consider the question 'what is critique?' along with the difference between critique, criticism and complaint; I argue for the need to understand in order to change, survive or leave; and, the intention of this book and its structure is set out.

In the previous chapter I outlined the genealogy of research on resilience. We saw that the early researchers understood resilience as a combination of both personal and environmental factors and brought ideas from child development and psychoanalysis to bear on its study. Subsequently other researchers tended to ignore the role of environment and concentrated attention instead on the study of personal characteristics that they claimed predicted various positive outcomes for individuals who have experienced adversity. Since then the concept has become increasingly individualized and popularly promoted as a set of behaviours that individuals can be taught and make an effort to adopt. Meanwhile other disciplines have taken up the idea of resilience and tried to apply it to ecological and other systems in a strong departure from the individualized approach that appears to predominate in psychology, or at least in much of its public presentation.

Resilience as wish fulfilment

In this chapter, I invite you to think about the outputs and theories of teams of scientists, not primarily as the products of objective disinterested procedures but to consider the work that goes on within scientific communities as unavoidably part of a cultural and political context. This context has an influence on the total scientific process, from the topics chosen to be investigated, through the very conceptualization and the imagination that occurs around this, to the perceived usefulness of solutions offered, the readiness of government and corporate bodies to fund and therefore promote particular streams of research and the pictures of preferred human subjectivity that underlie the entire process (i.e. healthiness is characterized by the autonomous and economically productive individual). Researchers rely on funders for their livelihoods and prestige. Some sociologists of science have investigated the constant entrepreneurial work that scientists do in order to sustain their laboratory (Latour 1987). Creating synergy between their own interests and the worldview and priorities of funders, whether they are state funders, corporations or major charities is a key to success for groups of scientists. It means that their research is likely to be the research that we hear about.

I will draw together the comments of writers who see the growing emphasis on resilience as the result of political forces, for example the preference of today's governments to focus on the positive and avoid costly attention to pathologies. There is, however, another related explanation for the attraction of resilience. As researcher James Anthony noted, the attractive story of the individual defeating and growing out of adversity has circulated in Western society for many centuries in the form of fairy tales, drama, novels and more recently in Hollywood films. It is a type of narrative that is so familiar that we do not realize that we know it. And it is not difficult to see that 'resilience' researchers and their funders also live and think within this zeitgeist. In fact, many researchers are frank about their optimistic and visionary ambitions as we saw in Chapter 1.

Some researchers give accounts of resilience where this cultural desirability is clear. For example, some case studies of apparently successful resilience seem to owe something to the American dream:[1]

> Sara was the youngest of four children raised in a dysfunctional family environment. Her father was an alcoholic and her mother was physically and verbally abusive. After years of fighting and yelling, Sara's parents ended up in a bitter and protracted divorce. Sara's needs were a low priority in the family chaos. Sara was a chubby baby, who turned into a chubby kid, who turned to food for most of her comfort. Despite her expanding waistline and often being the subject of cruel teasing, Sara knew she was smart as a whip and could always rely on her sense of humour to get her out of a tough situation. Sara had one best friend who lived down the street; her name was Jenny. Sara and Jenny shared everything: they conspired to grow

1 The term 'American dream' was first used by American historian James Truslow Adams in his book *The Epic of America* published in 1931 (http://america.day-dreamer.de/dream.htm). The 'dream' proposes a society where there is opportunity for all to achieve prosperity through hard work. In some versions it is individualistic and materialistic. Some say it covers over racism and lack of social mobility for the poor and for migrants. It has been fiercely parodied in Lars Von Trier's 2000 film *Dancer In The Dark* in which a Czech immigrant and single mother working in a factory in rural America is executed.

up and have fantastic lives. Sara was going to become a paediatrician and help sick children, get married, and have a perfect house with three kids. Meanwhile Sara's family continued to spiral down. They had stopped going to church, dropped out of the social functions they used to attend, and lost contact with family friends. Sara often found herself home alone or left at school until early evening, forgotten by her parents. Nonetheless, she did not bother to complain, tried to stay out of her parents' way, and generally took everything in stride. She dreamed of the day she would be off to college and medical school working hard to become a doctor. Sara grew up in that environment until she was 17. She did go off to college with a full academic scholarship. Once there she joined Jenny Craig, lost 60 pounds during her freshman year, and went on to enjoy social events and make new friends. She is a happy, practising paediatrician today.

(Earvolino-Ramirez 2007 p. 79)

In the above, not only do we see the fantasy story of the resilient individual promoted but the social values by which success is measured are also reinforced: friendship, family life, opportunity, education, hard work, professional success and being 'happy'. In some of the resilience literature it is hard to resist the conclusion that the researchers confuse normative social success with psychic health or rather see the former as evidence of the latter, i.e. if you are happily married with a good job then you must be psychologically well. Because of this it is easy to see how policymakers, funders and governments are attracted to resilience.

Resilience and 'responsibilization'

Many commentators have written about a style of government at work in many Western countries today. They tell us how governing (by which I mean the organization of society along with measures designed to bring about desirable outcomes usually economic but also behavioural) takes the form of placing responsibility on all individuals to avoid risk[2] and make the most of opportunities to maximize their health and independence (O'Malley 2009). The rather clumsy word used to describe this tendency is 'responsibilization'.[3] True to this observation we find the promoters of resilience interventions describing 'adversity' as 'risk' and the imperative to promote resilience through programmes aimed toward 'at-risk' groups on exactly these grounds:

> The growing knowledge base on resilience can be vital in guiding social policies to promote the well-being of disadvantaged, high-risk individuals in our society. The provision of treatment to children, adolescents and adults with mental disorders poses a great economic burden for society ... it is far more prudent to promote the development of resilient functioning as early as possible in the course

2 Risk is understood not as the operation of chance i.e. something like the roll of dice that cannot be foreseen and controlled but as something identified by professional researchers focussing on particular 'risky' populations e.g. we might assess the risk that a mental health patient poses to society by checking against a list of characteristics shown previously to be linked to danger. The list of factors might be added up to give a risk score and on this basis a decision made about whether to detain such a patient or allow them to go home (if they have one). These kinds of processes have to some extent replaced the judgement of professionals based on a more personal knowledge of the patient.

3 Here is a nice summary of the term from the book I have just cited:

> ... a term developed in the governmentality literature to refer to the process whereby subjects are rendered individually responsible for a task which previously would have been the duty of another – usually a state agency – or would not have been recognized as a responsibility at all. The process is strongly associated with neoliberal political discourses, where it takes on the implication that the subject being responsibilized [!] has avoided this duty or the responsibility has been taken away from them in the welfare-state era and managed by an expert or government agency.

of development than to implement treatment strategies designed to repair existing disorders among high-risk individuals . . .

(Luthar and Cicchetti 2000 p. 857)

The argument for interventions designed to promote resilience hinges on the use of the term 'modify'. If research has identified factors that appear to 'modify' the effect of adversity on the individual (high IQ, sense of humour for example) then interventions can be designed and delivered to at-risk groups to modify their behaviour further. I mentioned some studies that attempted this in the previous chapter.

Many researchers are keen to emphasize the individual variation in resilient behaviour; however, it seems that the identification of 'at-risk' groups (decided by the presence of various criteria e.g. parents with mental health problems, poverty) and the delivery of standardized interventions to these groups, rather than case by case support, does seem to negate the understanding of resilience as the particular individual's response to his or her given set of specific circumstances.

The focus of resilience is individualistic

As I mentioned in the last chapter, some resilience researchers, especially those with a commitment to social justice, have been at pains to distance their work – and the whole tradition – from simplistic ideas that resilience can be learned as a set of behaviours on the part of the individual irrespective of the context they find themselves in. They were concerned that the concept of resilience could be exploited by politicians and policymakers in order to reduce services to groups who would benefit from them. And there is plenty of evidence that the causes of health inequality are linked to structural factors in society (Marmot 2010). But today, despite these warnings, we are most likely to encounter talk of resilience in the form of advice about how to be more resilient by following certain tips, or should we say developing certain skills? Many on-line health based websites feature such 'self-help' guidance: in the US the American Psychological Association (see link below), the Mayo Clinic states:

> Test your resilience level and get tips to build your own resilience. . . . When something goes wrong, do you tend to bounce back or fall apart?
>
> (www.mayoclinic.org/tests-procedures/resilience-training/in-depth/resilience/art-20046311)

In the UK, Action for Happiness (www.actionforhappiness. org/10-keys-to-happier-living/find-ways-to-bounce-back/details) or The Happiness Foundation (www.thehappinessfoundation. co.uk/) are just a few of the examples available. Their guidance briefly acknowledges the importance of 'caring and supportive relationships' but the advice is, in a way that has become familiar, addressed to the individual. So even the place of supportive relationships is configured as an action that the individual must take to 'accept help and support' (www.apa.org/helpcenter/road-resilience.aspx) or by 'taking time to nurture our relationships' (www.actionforhappiness.org/10-keys-to-happier-living/find-ways-to-bounce-back/details).[4] The problem here is not that organizations have taken the time to publicize complex information (about the findings of resilience research) in an easily understood way but that ideas about resilience are distorted to fit into (or we could say to reproduce) an already established style and type of message that, in my view, has very limited real world usefulness. Imagine a continuum of communication: at one end is a brochure giving information about the signs and symptoms of cancer with advice about how to look for them and instructions about what to do if you think you find them.

---

4 In some cases (the Action for Happiness website) the terms resilience and resiliency are used interchangeably. Some resilience researchers have warned specifically against this on the grounds that these terms imply very different concepts.

At the other end is a romantic Hollywood love film – or an action movie if you prefer. Some promotion of resilience is nearer the Hollywood end. The point here is not that the brochure is based on science and the film is not. It is that some promotion of resilience (in the websites I have identified above, for example), like the many 'Ten habits of successful people' webpages, operates by repeating a kind of fantasy of human life[5] as does the Hollywood movie industry. In this fantasy people strive for a hazy fusion of individual qualities usually to do with healthiness, happiness, effectiveness and 'success' – in career or romantic terms (one of the resilience webpages says that resilience can lead to 'successful ageing' without explanation of what that might mean). This version of 'success' is underpinned by a kind of individualized capitalistic and bourgeois[6] version of the good life in which independence and responsibility for self are key features. The aim is to be motivational but often what underlies such pages is the promotion of the reputation of an individual or an organization along with, sometimes, its commercial products. At the same time some organizations rely on government funding for their work and because of this need to be seen to promote projects that align with that government's policies and priorities, the emphasis on 'happiness' for example (Wheeler 2014). The tough social and political challenges of resilience have been turned into encouragements to the population to try to be more optimistic and cope better or to search for the benefits (not in the welfare sense of course) of adversity. Despite the nods toward the argument that good relationships or being 'part of a faith community' are components of resilience, the net effect of the proliferation of these messages is the reinforcement of a picture of a society made up of individuals each working hard to maximize their individual potential. Resilience is co-opted into this project.

5   Usually by hiring journalists or content writers to provide this specific genre of work.
6   See Chapters 6 and 8.

Critiques of resilience from radical social justice

Not far from the world of nursing, resilience, along with ideas of recovery and strengths, has been evoked as an empowering new emphasis for those with mental health diagnoses. Some have argued that while this looks like good news for these patients and 'ex-patients', survivors, it covers over the continuing power of professional authority (to deliver prescribed CBT for example) and the failure of societies to take responsibility for the fact that some mental health issues are at least partly the result of, or exacerbated by, social injustice and societal unfairness. Examples given are depression among women and schizophrenia among Afro-Caribbean men.

> As for resilience, the concept parallels the notion of recovery. Where recovery posits the ability of subjects to recover from an illness, the notion of resilience ostensibly recognizes the innate capacities of people to 'bounce back' in the face of challenges or sources of distress. The capacity to be resilient is not, however, left to chance: psychologists have become authorities in instilling resilience, especially through the increasingly authoritative techniques such as cognitive behavioural therapy, or 'positive psychology'. These changes are deeply tied to broader austerity measures: getting citizens to be resilient in the face of challenges is not only cheap (in that it diverts patients out of public health care systems, in favour of self-help and positive thinking), it is also about aspiring to create a resilient citizenry, able to cope with uncertainty. This is a technology of looking inward: rather than confronting austerity measures or other matters of social justice through political action, citizens are enjoined to look inward, gather their strengths, and be resilient. Recovery and resilience, then, are notions deeply embedded with both the economic and the social imperatives of contemporary neoliberalism.
>
> (Howell and Voronka 2012 p. 4)

Some critiques of resilience focus on its possible attractiveness to politicians because of its focus on positives and solutions rather than on problems. Mark Neocleous suggests:

> 'Resilience' has in the last decade become one of the key political categories of our time. It falls easily from the mouths of politicians, a variety of state departments are funding research into it, urban planners are now obliged to take it into consideration, and academics are falling over themselves to conduct research on it.
>
> (Neocleous 2013 p. 3)

Is the argument for resilience circular?

My next critique of resilience research stems from a suspicion, when reading this kind of work, that arguments about the character and operation of resilience are circular. I think there are three ways in which this occurs. Researchers start to use the term 'resilience' to attempt to give an evocative or metaphorical name to the puzzling observation that some individuals seem less permanently damaged by adversity than others.[7] They then look for the components or predictors of this phenomenon, termed protective if they are positive, and vulnerability factors if they seem to predispose the individual to damage. They then argue that the operation of these factors leads to an outcome when the individual is faced with adversity in terms of a collection of observable behaviours the presence of which shows the presence of resilience while their relative absence shows that

---

7 Perhaps the earlier term 'invulnerable' reflected the fact that a generation of child psychologists grew up reading Superman comics. (Among the attributes that made Superman who he was, was his invulnerability. You could try to crush him under weights but he would always survive. It would be inaccurate to say that Superman 'bounced back'. That was left to fellow super-hero Bouncing Boy who perhaps better embodied the contemporary idea of resilience. Wikipedia informs us that he had 'Limited invulnerability (while bouncing) and resistance to injury' https://en.wikipedia.org/wiki/Bouncing_Boy).

the individual is not resilient. Could we not argue that 'resilience' is simply a metaphorical label used to conveniently talk about the observable result of the operation of a number of factors (such as intelligence, consistent parenting) for the individual? The conventional account of scientific research is that a pre-existing phenomenon comes to the attention of scientists who then go on to investigate its components using the measuring instruments that they have to hand and discover what it is made of or what causes it. However it is just as plausible to say that scientists agree to define or construct something as existing when their measuring instruments show certain readings.[8] In this case those readings are 'measures' (very often individuals' own self-description) of the amount of intelligence or of 'good natured, easy temperament' at play with, or 'possessed by' a particular individual. So the concept, or construct, of resilience does not *explain* why some individuals seem less permanently damaged by adversity than others. Resilience is not a kind of good that you can obtain in a market. It is simply the label applied to describe the outcome of the operation of an array of characteristics and contextual features. We could go one step further and say that those characteristics and contextual features are themselves just other constructs devised through the agreement of the same or a similar group of scientists in order to get their work done and talk conveniently to one another.[9] It is when any of these terms escape the confines of the lab or the scientific

8 This kind of argument that questions what is happening in the process of scientific discovery is summarized in the slim but radically subversive *Science: The Very Idea* by Steve Woolgar (1988).

9 I am thinking, loosely, of the argument made by post-structuralists, for example Jacques Derrida in the (1982) essay *Différance* argues that it is impossible to nail down the meaning of any signifier without simply using other signifiers. According to Ferdinand de Saussure any linguistic sign, which he saw as made of two components, the signifier – the acoustic event – and the signified – the concept or mental construct, only has meaning because of its difference to other signifiers, so there is no final meaning outside of the system of signifiers. A readable introduction to Saussure's theories is found in *The Continental Philosophy Reader* (eds Kearney and Rainwater 1996 pp. 291–304).

conference and end up somewhere on the fringes of the public domain, for example on the website of Action for Happiness, that managers, policymakers and general enthusiasts start to believe that they really exist.

A second type of circularity is at work in some studies of nurses. In these studies nurses are asked by researchers to talk about or to rate themselves in relation to resilience. In other words they are presented the concept of resilience and then by discussing it simply reinforce the researcher's belief in the crucial role of resilience. It is possible to substitute a range of other terms, such as 'job satisfaction', into nurses' talk in this kind of study without losing any meaning. Sometimes, also, the assumed direction of the action of resilience could easily be reversed, for example when nurses produce resilient talk, this could be the effect of a conducive and perhaps specialist environment, with particular resources, rather than any pre-existing personal attribute. Some research acknowledges that certain environments can foster conditions that appear to enable features of resilience. This includes an organization of work that enables staff to maintain long-term, meaningful relationships with residents [in an aged care facility] (Cameron and Brownie 2010), or that settings with high peer cohesion and good educational support can foster aspects of resilience (Gillespie *et al.* 2009). If resilience were purely a matter of individual disposition how can we explain whole organizations or units that appear to descend into poor care? Did they not recruit any resilient people?

There is a third type of circularity to be detected in nursing research on resilience in the form of the tendency of some nursing papers to draw on other nursing papers for their understanding of the concept of resilience, occasionally making no reference at all to any studies beyond this field of work, ignoring the key debates in the 'mainstream' literature and repeating a sometimes partial or distorted version of resilience. Often this results in a picture of resilience as a kind of nursing competency to be developed and demonstrated by practitioners. I also see the dangerous assumption that social status can be read off as evidence of resilience. Those who leave nursing are those who lacked resilience while those who stay show that they have it.

So is resilience any use?

This is a good point at which to summarize the argument of the book so far. For a number of reasons, talk and promotion of resilience has come to the fore globally, in the West, in the UK and in nursing in today's NHS. The notion has recent origins in research into child development and the relationship between an individual child and their environment. This complex concept has been simplified, first among the so-called 'psy' professions[10] many of which are predominantly more interested in working at an individual level and less orientated to social issues, by an increasing focus on 'internal' characteristics and skills. Second, we could say resilience has been distorted or even exploited by those who realize that it can be co-opted into the 'responsibiliza-tion' that some commentators believe characterizes the kind of society we find ourselves in today. From this point of view it becomes part of a move, to put it crudely but accurately, to reduce investment in welfare. Finally, it has been taken up in nursing with the hope that it might ease the experience of hard-pressed nurses. However I believe that much of the research and interventions around resilience by nurses are haunted by a sense of powerlessness and pessimism about dealing with the issues that make the apparent need for resilience so urgent in the first place. That is one reason that they tend to be so individually based. When a situation is intolerable, coping and resilience is not a good answer.

Help, why shouldn't I build up resilience?

To paraphrase Catch Van Jones, a social and environmental justice activist and advisor to the White House: the problem with

---

10 I am thinking of the term 'psy-complex' used by some writers to describe the set of professions that claim to be dealing with the human soul, the psyche: psychology, psychiatry, psychoanalysis, psychotherapy, psychiatric nursing and psychiatric social work. The term comes from the work of Michel Foucault and others who analysed the part played by the 'psy' professions in regulating family life, sexuality, the mind and rationality.

resilience thinking is often that it's about – whoever you are – if something bad happens, we want you to be able to bounce back to where you were. What if where you were sucks? (Helper 2015). Much talk about resilience in adults focuses on dealing with traumatic events in the shape, for example, of the death of a loved one, a terminal diagnosis or a personal attack. Once these events have occurred perhaps the challenge is to learn how to respond positively and grow from these traumas. Resilience in the workplace is very different. I pointed out earlier that resilience researchers in nursing have listed a number of causes of stress and adversity: high turnover, political change, under-resourcing of public healthcare, casualization, staff shortages, bullying, abuse and violence. These all exist for particular reasons. Often they are the result of particular decisions or on-going strategies devised by particular groups, such as saving on an organization's staffing budget in order to apply for Foundation Trust status. Who is likely to suffer the most from such policies? Perhaps the groups that make the least trouble.[11] One website says 'resilience is being able to roll with the punches'. I think it is preferable to make sure you stop getting hit rather than learn how to be able to last longer before you finally collapse.

There is another argument that nurses who have some personal resilience abilities are those who are more likely to be confident enough to act assertively, perhaps to challenge and change what is unacceptable in their environments and to protect themselves – so for the individual nurse, surely there can be no harm in learning these skills and aptitudes? That could be true; however, I find no evidence or mention of this in any of the research on nurses and resilience and most child development

---

11 As I write this, I have just heard that the UK government has conceded to the demands of the BMA (British Medical Association – the doctors' trade union) regarding the introduction of a new working hours contract. They did this because junior doctors threatened to, and were about to strike. Health Secretary Jeremy Hunt backed down on the evening before the day of the planned strike. See www.theguardian.com/politics/2015/nov/30/doctors-strike-jeremy-hunt-announces-potential-agreement-with-bma. The conflict is not over however.

researchers emphasize that resilience is as much a feature of the environment as the child's characteristics and that interventions that do not include attention to the environment are unlikely to have lasting benefits.

It's decision time: what are the alternatives?

Here are three things you can do as a nurse in today's tough NHS (or other complex and pressured environments): you can understand the causes of day-to-day problems, challenge and fight for change perhaps as a trade union activist or by working to move into positions of power, you can leave and bring a staffing crisis and policy change perhaps one step nearer or you can stay and develop appreciation and gratitude for what you have, along with optimism that one day things might get better.[12]

An alternative: critical resilience

The argument for educating nurses in the UK and elsewhere in the world at degree level is that nursing work is complex and needs people who have high levels of knowledge and analytical abilities, and are able to confidently debate options with colleagues from other professions and make sophisticated decisions. Usually this ability is understood as applying to clinical tasks and aspects of patient management but the influences on nursing work and healthcare come from many directions. Analytical abilities might be turned to questions like 'Why is this unit under-resourced?', 'What is the effect of healthcare reorganization on discharging our patients on time?', 'Why do nurses from my background seem to be passed over when it comes to promotion?' For me the key difference between resilience and 'critical resilience' is that critical resilience is about understanding ourselves and our experiences in relation to our society – to take a phrase from feminist consciousness-raising

12 There is a fourth alternative, which is to become cynical. If you work with someone who has taken this route you will see that it brings with it some kind of satisfaction. But it has a cost.

groups (Chicago Women's Liberation Union 1970). The combination of becoming informed about the political and policy forces acting on day-to-day working experience and frank, mutually supportive discussion can develop critical resilience. Neither on its own is enough. Getting informed by reading a radical nursing blog on health policy or on the latest Nursing and Midwifery Council (NMC) initiative for example is just the starting point for responding. And discussion without information can too easily turn into complaint where the pleasure is not in the creative energy released by analysis and planning to do something but in repeating expressions of suffering. So, getting together and getting informed are the first steps in developing critical resilience.

It has been my discovery that things in life are not what they seem. Or perhaps, to put it another way, the discovery is that things are how they are for particular reasons. Usually we are kept busy – and if we are fortunate interested – working for the things we need. We rarely take the time to look closely at our world from any particular perspective. Added to that the

Seeing that we are talking about complaint, I invite you to critique complaint as an experiment to try out yourself. This could mark the first steps in what I am proposing is the route of critical resilience.

Next time you are in a group of colleagues or fellow students, listen out for when the conversation moves into 'complaint'. Make a note of the features of this kind of talk. Here are some suggested questions to ask yourself:

Is there enjoyment in this talk? If so what is it attached to?
Is there energy? If so where does it arise?
How accurate are the speakers about what they are
    speaking about?
Do some kinds of comment get squashed?
What is the outcome of the talk?

status quo also offers us some sweeteners – position, identity, a paycheque in return for our compliance. But unless we wake up to the forces influencing how things are as they are we will be vulnerable to a kind of befogged powerlessness. I will spell this out further in Chapter 7.

What is critique and how is it different from 'criticism' or 'complaint'?

The notion of critique is easy to misunderstand, so let's clear the ground before we go further. Critique can be both an activity and the product of that activity. Here is a definition of the activity: to critique is 'to evaluate (a theory or a practice) in a detailed and analytical way' and this produces, not surprisingly, 'a detailed analysis and assessment of something, often a literary piece or a philosophical or political theory'. I have taken the following simple summary of the 'difference between criticism and critique' from a book about setting up support groups for those starting out writing fiction and poetry. It is aimed at reassuring those worried about exposing their work to others but is still a good start for us:

The difference between criticism and critique:

Criticism finds fault/Critique looks at structure

Criticism looks for what's lacking/Critique finds what's working

Criticism condemns what it doesn't understand/Critique asks for clarification

Criticism is spoken with a cruel wit and sarcastic tongue/ Critique's voice is kind, honest, and objective

Criticism is negative/Critique is positive (even about what isn't working)

Criticism is vague and general/Critique is concrete and specific

Criticism has no sense of humour/Critique insists on laughter, too

Criticism looks for flaws in the writer as well as the writing/ Critique addresses only what is on the page.

(Reeves 2002)

These simple dichotomies work well in the context of literary criticism and make the point to us that while criticism can be characterized as negative in intent and style, critique is a practice that demands a rigorous engagement with its object. It is also productive because it can lead to action. If the fleeting and perverse pleasure of criticism sometimes lies in the real or imagined humiliation of another, the energy and enjoyment in critique is in understanding, for example, the connection between apparently unconnected events, the hidden history of an apparently self-evident truth, the internal contradiction within a government or professional policy, and the reality of one's situation within a system. While acknowledging that critique can on occasion become flavoured with a taste of negativity, I hope it is clear by now that the two have little in common.

The third of my 'Three Cs' is complaint – the topic of my proposed first critical thought experiment above. I have my own theories about complaint in nursing and I will summarize them with just enough detail to distinguish this traditional nursing pastime from the practice of critique. Everybody complains and every occupation complains about its particular predicament during coffee breaks – in those jobs where workers are lucky enough to have them. But complaint in nursing has a couple of specific characteristics that I think are a result of its particular history and make it unusual. Here is the outline of my argument.

1   Nursing promotes an idealized vision of nursing work along with the identity of the nurse as fully caring and fully autonomous (see Chapter 5). However, this kind of idealized practice is impossible partly for organizational reasons but partly because of resistance 'internal' to nurses themselves as work with patients generates high amounts of anxiety (Menzies 1960).

2   Faced with an everyday experience that is strongly at odds with this idealized vision, nurses look to external constraints for an explanation. They do this because this provokes less anxiety than profoundly questioning a fundamental ideology of autonomous caring in nursing.

3   In addition to this, there is a particular kind of pleasure found by nurses in repeating accounts of their apparently powerless position. According to some writers, feeling one's self to be a righteous victim can provide a sense of having 'moral high ground' (Žižek 2005).

4   This pleasure in powerlessness, and willingness to be 'flexible' or do your duty in spite of the personal cost is a feature of nursing that is essential for its functioning within the highly pressured structures of healthcare. It reinforces acquiescence among the workforce making it susceptible to drift into poor practice instead of resistance.[13] It also makes it possible for the workforce to be exploited by governments and management hard-pressed to make a straining health system work.

It should be clear by now that my feeling about complaint in nursing is that while it may be understandable it is in the end unproductive. We can even see the pleasure that nurses seem to gain in complaint as an example of what Freud called the death drive (Freud [1920] 1984), part of a compulsive repetition among those who have undergone trauma, of the traumatic event.[14] In this case the trauma is of having to manage the suffering of patients but lacking the power, for organizational and other reasons, to act as they believe is necessary. Work psychologists call this high demand low control work (Karasek *et al.* 1998).

I want to end this section on the difference between critique and criticism and complaint by introducing another of those C-words. I want to suggest that critique can even open the way to compassion. First imagine some kind of dyadic situation – just you and another nurse for example. You can imagine whatever you like about who they are and what they want and,

13   This summary is based on work I did with a psychoanalyst and is published in *Nursing Philosophy* Traynor and Evans (2014).

14   On the opening page of my favourite nursing blog, Grumbling Appendix, a commenter writes that she expects that there is a lot to complain about [in nursing work]. Grumbling Appendix replies 'Let's not call it complaining. Let's say it's more "intelligent critique!"' (https://grumblingappendix.wordpress.com/about/).

if the nurse in question is a manager, what they want of you. If you introduce a third term you can escape this possibly claustrophobic situation (think of the infinite reflections you see when standing between two mirrors). The third term is a structure or theory i.e. a critique that you can apply from outside this dyad to explain the situation and the behaviour of that other nurse, or any other healthcare worker, university tutor, etc. So critique can free you from blaming individuals when structural explanations give you a possible insight into why another person might behave as they do. Here is a diagram to put this idea even more simply.

Nurse → critique → compassion

In this chapter we have covered a lot of ground. I have set out some critiques of research on resilience and, more importantly, of the way that this research has been attractive to governments and co-opted into a culture that is highly individualized. I have suggested that its take up in nursing research suffers the same individualizing tendency. 'Resilience' works as an enigmatic signifier, that is as a kind of empty placeholder that different groups use in ways that are familiar to them and can further their interests. Finally I have introduced a concept that I think is more useful and called this 'critical resilience'. I have set out the difference between critique and other more familiar activities. I have suggested that you explore the possibility of setting up groups with your fellow students or colleagues to develop informed critiques about aspects of your working life.

Chapter 3

How compassionate are you?

JIMMY (second-year mental health branch student): Well, on paper, nurses are supposed to be compassionate, they're supposed to have empathy, be sensitive, caring and all that, but do we have all these qualities in one person, to be able to be called a good nurse? That is another question.

MICHAEL: What do other people think?

NANCY: It's about who you are and the manner in which you treat your family or somebody else is the manner you should go and treat a patient and we can't all have all these qualities but you use what you have. . . . I think it's just – the thing is who you are from within, it's not something that is taught. I can learn about medication and everything else but for me to be a nurse, for me to have it within me, it's me in a way, I don't know, it has to be.

In this chapter I ask where today's emphasis on compassion in nursing came from; I discuss the uses and abuses of the idea and whether compassion could be a red herring in nursing work. Compassion is a kind of disciplinary term and the workforce is recruited and probed to make sure they have enough of it. By looking at research on professional socialization I discuss the possibility that idealism can lead to disenchantment. The chapter also draws on a recent reframing of so-called compassion failure as a psychological phenomenon associated with highly pressured contexts. I go even further by questioning the nature and attraction of empathy. As a solution I discuss alternatives to compassion – these concern a combination of carefully listening to patients and high levels of professional knowledge.

If you apply to train as a nurse in the UK today the chances are that at some point you will be asked to attend an interview. The first question you will have to answer is likely to be about the qualities that you believe you have that will make you a good nurse. And the expectation for interviewer and applicant alike seems to be that answers will feature compassion, or a caring nature, as the number one quality that will make a good nurse. In this chapter I would like to investigate where this taken for granted assumption came from and some of the problems that it brings to practising nurses.

As a thought experiment either imagine or with a friend or colleague re-enact your last interview (either for a student place or a job interview) where you were asked this, or a very similar question. In this imaginary, no-pressure re-enactment try telling 'the truth' and see what this reveals to you about yourself and your assumptions as well as the profession's assumptions about the 'right' answer. Here are a few possible answers to the question:

I think you need to be highly intelligent to be a nurse – I am highly intelligent.

I had an experience of terrible nursing care with my father/mother/child/close friend and I vowed to get into the profession and prove it could be done better.

I want a professional job where I get responsibility, respect and a good salary.

I'm not sure that I do want to be a nurse but I want to try it out and see if it works for me.

Why compassion? Why now?

Surprisingly, in their introductory advice for someone thinking about a career in nursing neither NHS Careers (http://nursing.nhscareers.nhs.uk/why) nor the Royal College of Nursing (wwww.rcn.org.uk/professional-development/become-a-nurse) highlight compassion as a prime quality. Instead these organizations emphasize leadership qualities, technical competence and decision-making ability after the filter of basic numeracy and literacy abilities.[1] So why is talk of compassion, along with its apparent synonyms caring and empathy so all-pervasive in and around nursing and why do so many of those who want to enter the profession feel it would be hazardous not to mention it?

To think about this question we need to take a similar approach to the investigation of resilience that I offered in Chapter 1. Here we need to consider how nursing was shaped in influential ways at particular moments and in particular kinds of culture. To do this I am going to first spend time in late nineteenth-century Britain, then journey over to 1980s United States, then return to the UK in time to hear the Chief Nursing Officer for England talking about the six Cs.

Modern nursing was produced in the peculiar culture of nineteenth-century Britain where respectable women did not go out to work, the country's universities only admitted men and only men could vote.[2] I will talk in more detail about nursing's history in Chapter 5. I will mention here that to develop and present nursing as a viable occupation for women required considerable skill on the part of those promoting it to avoid the suspicion of patriarchal society in general and condemnation from medical men with whom nurses would have to work in particular. In a society preoccupied by the dangers of immoral sexual behaviour and the need to control all opportunities for its eruption, women were given a restricted repertoire of roles and identities. Aside from the stereotype of the 'fallen woman', the role of women from affluent backgrounds was to provide order to the home as a domestic moral guardian leaving public

---

1 The Nursing and Midwifery Council include 'Care, compassion and communication' in their list of five groups of essential skills that universities have to include in all pre-registration nursing courses.

2 A great deal has been written about nursing's roots in the Victorian era. See for example any of this small selection: McGann (1992), Rafferty (1993), Baly (1995), Rafferty (1996).

life by and large to men. It is no surprise that figures such as Florence Nightingale, herself a prominent exception to this convention, took pains to describe nursing work and women's social progress in terms of duty, calling and desire to serve (McDonald 2005). Neither is it a surprise to learn that preparation for this profession was highly disciplined with a strong focus on character training.

As the twentieth century arrived and the basis for nursing work became more technical than moral and with the influence of the feminism of the mid-century, nursing's subordinate relationship to medicine became uncomfortable. Prominent leaders in the profession, particularly in the United States, began to search for ways to differentiate nursing from its more powerful, and then largely male, neighbouring profession. This project took many forms. Some believed that nursing needed its own scientific knowledge base that would differentiate it as an autonomous profession. Some rejected the entire paradigm of scientific knowledge and argued instead that nursing should develop according to a distinctive female way of knowing (Hagell 1989). Some wished to elevate the importance of nursing by claiming that nursing practice was an ethical activity and a vital part of human evolution (Paterson and Zderad 1976, Benner and Wrubel 1989, Benner *et al.* 1996). Nursing leaders, faced perhaps with the limited sphere of the profession's autonomy in most healthcare systems made the very most of the possibilities that nurses had for action. Identification with the patient's interests and the claim of a moral high ground led to phrases and slogans along the lines of 'nurses are the patient's advocate' and 'doctors cure, nurse care'.[3] The trouble with such slogans

---

3 This phrase of unknown origin has been particularly troublesome. Buresh and Gordon (2006) for example, see its repetition by nurses as an unhelpful denial of nurses' curative work perpetuating the exaggerated valuing by the public of medical work within patient care. An alternative view is that nurses adopt this shorthand to give moral value to their work in the face of well-established medical professional status and influence. For a provocative critique of how nurses participate in what Nietzsche called 'slave morality' regarding the elevation of caring see John Paley's (2002) paper on this topic.

is that their repetition can stand in for thinking and feed into an often sentimental view of nurses held by sections of the public and some political leaders (Hallam 2000). The result has been that nurses generally identify themselves with caring and the ambiguity of the term – the word can mean anything from performing physical procedures to something morally loaded, associated with compassion and close to loving – is sometimes reflected in the ambiguity of the claim. 'I perform acts of care' can easily drift to 'I am a caring person'. To the question 'Why do you think you would make a good nurse?' it becomes natural to reply, 'Because I am a caring person'.

With this strong identification with a moral orientation, the fall from grace threatened by a series of scandals during the 2010s that involved nurses was all the more shocking. The most discussed were the events at Stafford Hospital where it was reported that elderly patients were neglected by nursing staff. However further failures appeared in the UK media (BBC Panorama 2011) and in government-commissioned reports (Keogh 2013). The public responded with outrage and incredulity at these apparently widespread acts of cruelty. The final report into the events at Stafford was published in February 2013 (Francis 2013b). The report identified the complex causes of poor medical and nursing care detailing how the pressures on working culture from management led to atrocious failures of care delivery. The report claimed that entrants to nursing were not adequately prepared to resist the challenges of working in such NHS cultures which tolerated poor standards. The Francis proposal was that: 'There should be an increased focus in nurse training, education and professional development on the practical requirements of delivering compassionate care in addition to the theory' (Section 23.49 p. 1513). The report also proposed that prospective student nurses should complete time in health care support roles as an introduction to caring work and as a trial to exclude those unfitted for such work. In addition, the report recommended the selection of applicants who could 'demonstrate possession of' the values, attitudes and behaviour appropriate for the profession (p. 1513). Of the report's 290 recommendations, those which were most apparently straightforward to put into practice were the most likely to be backed by politicians.[4] The profession, clearly under government pressure even before the final report was published intensified its identification with caring and compassion. The Chief Nursing Officer (CNO) for England published the document Compassion in Practice (Commissioning Board Chief Nursing Officer and DH Chief Nursing Adviser 2012) involving the launch of the 'six Cs' alongside action plans aimed at safeguarding standards of patient care. This included a call for recruitment to be based on applicant 'values' as well as technical skills.

With these challenges to nursing's previously positive public standing and the re-emergence of calls from certain quarters for nurse education to return to those unpretentious School of Nursing days, the Royal College of Nursing (RCN) commissioned Lord Willis to conduct an inquiry into pre-registration nursing education in the UK, specifically how it might create and maintain a workforce of 'competent, compassionate' nurses prepared to deliver services into the future' (Willis 2012 p. 4). The ease with which these two terms are coupled gives a strong foretaste of the report's conclusion. Counter to the sometimes circulating misogynistic belief that too much education for nurses damages their caring instincts, the Report found no evidence of this peculiar inverse relationship. On the whole, it stated, better-qualified nurses are associated with better patient outcomes.

Meanwhile, the Department of Health issued instructions (the Mandate) to Health Education England (Department of Health

---

4 The prospect of decoupling the government's ultimate command and control over the NHS from the responses of managers under pressure when healthcare represents such a substantial proportion of government spending would be a vast challenge to the imagination. Issuing instructions to nursing to sharpen up its recruitment is far less challenging, and many MPs and their constituents may have been sceptical of nursing's degree pretensions all along.

5 HEE is the body that at the time of writing is funded by the Department of Health (£4,930 million in 2014/5) to commission and oversee the education of the healthcare workforce in England. The way of funding nurse education is set to change to a system of student loans. Implications for HEE (not to mention recruitment and workforce planning) are unclear.

2013)[5] to introduce measures intended to address the 'failures of care' highlighted in the Francis report. This involved requiring Health Education England (HEE) to ensure that its recruitment, selection and training should promote particular values and behaviour among the NHS workforce. Perhaps rather optimistically, progress was to be assessed by changes in scores from patient surveys on staff behaviour and the 'family and friends' test. The short section in the Mandate on Values and Behaviours (p. 13) also included the requirement for HEE to set up and evaluate pilot schemes for prospective nursing students to work for up to a year as healthcare assistants at no additional cost. HEE in turn commissioned consultants Work Psychology Group to look at current evidence on effective ways to do 'values-based recruitment' (Health Education England 2014). The group's review starts by teasing apart the different concepts of values, personality, motivation and behaviour and describing the highly complex and contextual relationship between them. The constant reference point in the DH mandate, the resulting HEE documents and the commissioned review of recruitment and values is the Francis report, yet the Francis diagnosis of what went wrong and why problems at Stafford were not identified sooner is extremely broad. It ranges from behaviour and policy from the Department of Health interpreted locally as bullying, constant NHS reorganization, regulatory gaps, through misguided senior management actions, ineffective organizational communication systems, organizational defensiveness and secrecy to cultural tolerance of poor standards (Francis 2013a pp. 65–6). It is hard to resist the suspicion that the political need to be seen to act has driven a costly series of initiatives focussing on recruit-ment where the benefit is likely to be tangential. The array of political and policy forces that act on NHS staff – unwanted reorganizations, directives seen as bullying, relentless drives for cost-saving – are left, more or less, as they are. With the requirement for values based recruitment a few unsuitable potential nurses may be directed away from the NHS but the rest who are motivated to put patient care at the centre of their attention will still be challenged by immersion in stressed and dysfunctional environments. Many commentators have argued that the problems with NHS failures do not lie primarily in the poor values of those entering the service but with what culture and context does to even the most highly motivated individuals. Later in this chapter I will summarize one of the most powerful critiques that takes this approach.

As we saw with the drive for resilience, the political and structural causes of NHS problems remain relatively ignored. In the case of values, a solution is proposed or rather required by government, taken up by policymakers, invested in by implementers, researchers are hired to investigate it and the individual and their deficiencies becomes the focus for attention. To return to the beginning of this chapter, when you applied to train as a nurse, or for your most recent job, those assessing you will have been obliged, whether they believed in its usefulness or not, to devise a selection process designed to reveal your 'values' in order to assess your suitability for nursing work. This is not new for employers and universities but the type of obligation is (see following box).

Values-based recruitment in action: At a recent meeting that I attended with a local Clinical Commissioning Group we were given a presentation by two members of a recruitment company. Being ahead of their competitors they had been working on a way of helping the NHS deliver on its obligation to practise 'values-based recruitment'. The company had built a website and a smart phone app that set up a range of questions (I think there were between 6 and 10) that job applicants had to work through before the interview and send the result to the company from their phone. At the click of a button the managers who were doing the recruiting could discover the overall psychological profile for each applicant and be given a series of predetermined 'personalized' questions to ask at interview in order to probe areas which the system considered potentially problematic aspects of the applicant's profile. While some around the table were sceptical, the NHS managers present were clearly attracted by the product. What they liked, I think, was that with the payment to this company they could 'tick the box' for values-based recruitment for their entire organization and then possibly move on to deal with another in a series of urgent imperatives that piled up on their desks.

What happens to nurses who care?

As we have seen, the idea of caring for patients has become central to nursing's identity, as much to those outside the profession as those familiar with the technical and organizational skills needed to actually do the job. But students and new nurses seem to have a different relationship to caring from their more experienced colleagues. In this section I want to talk about some of the research done into this topic in order to show how counter-intuitive some of the conclusions are. I argue that for students and newly qualified nurses understanding how healthcare is delivered is perhaps more important than either being caring or the type of resilience we saw in Chapter 1.

Professional socialization is usually understood as a process that involves new entrants learning the behaviour, norms, skills, attitudes and values of a profession.[6] Key to this process is the 'internalization' of these features in a way that gradually constitutes professional identity. Formal training enables much of this learning but it is widely acknowledged that informal learning, some of it in the form of responses to the workplace, is an integral and less controllable aspect of professional

---

6 A recent review on the topic of socialization commissioned by the RCN (2015) starts with this succinct definition of professional socialization: Socialization refers to the process by which a person acquires skills, knowledge and identity characteristic of a profession (www.rcn.org.uk/ development/practice/professional_attitudes_and_behaviours/socialisation).

socialization. Early research on socialization of medical students, most notably the study *Boys in White* by Howard Becker and colleagues published in the early 1960s (Becker *et al.* 1961), shows how students' sense of fear and vulnerability, for example of being discovered by senior doctors to have messed up on a lab test, drives their behaviour toward their overall goal of becoming qualified. The process of socialization involves the taking to pieces of new recruits' lay identity (how a lay person would understand events and act), often traumatically, and the building up of a convincing professional identity during training. In looking at the process that nursing students go through I want to focus on the suggestion that vulnerability and fear are essential mechanisms of socialization rather than unfortunate and avoidable side effects. I warned that this would be counter-intuitive.

Research into socialization of nursing students gives a clear message about the disorientation experienced by students and the dissonance that results for them. The elements that go to make up this dissonance vary from study to study as I am about to show. I want to point out, however, that sometimes the 'lay understanding' of students is identified by the researchers themselves with the profession's highest values and that this is in contrast to other studies done either in medicine or into nursing by researchers from outside the profession. An early nurse researcher into this topic was Kath Melia (1987). She believed students experienced dissonance between classroom and practice versions of nursing. Other researchers considered that the dissonance was between what they term professional idealism and practice realism (Mackintosh 2006, Curtis *et al.* 2012). For example, Curtis and colleagues investigated what 19 student nurses at one university thought about the value of compassionate care and their own ability to be able to deliver this once they were qualified. The authors appear to agree with the students who they studied in considering that it was the context of care delivery which imposes constraints on what participants describe as being empathetic, holistic and doing what is right for the patient. The students identified time pressures and rapid patient throughput as frustrating their desire to be involved in these kinds of 'compassionate' activities. The personal satisfaction that these students wished for is identified with professional nursing ideals by the students as well as the authors while any constraints are pictured as coming from outside the profession, from the effects of government policy and organizational ways of working. The authors described the students as having a sense of vulnerability in the face of constraints beyond their control and as being concerned about reconciling two conflicting desires – to 'fit in' in the workplace and to maintain their initial idealism.

Other researchers (Greenwood 1993, Mackintosh 2006) believe socialization can lead to desensitization of students. Mackintosh saw her student participants falling into two groups by the end of training: those who completely rejected the apparent failure to care that they had witnessed among staff during their training and those who recognized that some degree of emotional desensitization was essential to preserve themselves in a work environment that was often distressing. She summarized her participants' dichotomy as between 'working from the heart' and not 'bursting into tears every time somebody dies' (p. 958).

Another team investigated the effect of experience and time on the idealism of newly qualified nurses (Maben *et al.* 2007). Jill Maben and her colleagues interviewed nurses in their last year of study in 3 UK universities, shortly after they qualified and again 3 years after qualification. By the end of the study she classified three types of nurse: sustained idealists, compromised idealists and crushed idealists. Within the study the explicit transmission of nursing's values is seen as the domain of the university classroom. But the practice setting, in contrast, is the site of informal learning where destructive 'covert rules' (p. 103) are at work. The nurses in the study understand the need for these rules as an effect of the intrusive managerialist and high-pressured environments that today's nurses are compelled to work within. In the light of these findings, Maben and colleagues suggest that the profession's strong orientation to the delivery of care to individuals may be out of date at a time when nursing work is often supervisory.

The message from *Boys in White* is that professional social-ization can be seen as largely successful because it enables the profession to continue to function with some stability – new recruits do not leave, they know how to behave and the public continue to trust them. Much of the nursing research, by contrast, concludes that socialization is a major problem because students and new recruits are presented as *starting out* as identifying with the profession's proper 'ideals' but as *losing* this as they qualify and continue to work in the profession. This points to a surprising inversion, which is possibly an effect of the researchers in nursing generally being nurses themselves and identifying, consciously or unconsciously, with these values whereas Becker and others are not members of the group they are studying.

What I want to emphasize from this brief look at socialization and care and compassion is that most of those who enter nursing change as they are forced to reassess their outsider view of what nursing work is like. As most researchers tell us, socialization is a total learning experience and not just a cognitive education. New nurses can be shaken to the core by their experiences. The combination of the trauma of illness and dying and what can feel like, or actually be, unsympathetic work environments makes the new nurse susceptible to unfamiliar ways of responding and behaving. As a new nurse you may be hoping for one-to-one relationships with your patients[7] but instead you are confronted with a dozen or more patients all making demands on your care and attention. Whether it is out of self-protection or simply to get through the work, you are likely to measure your emotional investment in any individual patient encounter more con-sciously than you perhaps thought you would. Your experienced colleagues will have learned this long ago but they will manage this with the share of intelligence, self-awareness and under-standing of the system that each possesses. What you find you need is not so much compassion but resilience.

---

7 Some believe that the fusion and sense of oneness of a baby and its mother sets the unconscious model for all of life's subsequent relationships. (This kind of relationship is uncompromisingly dyadic – and unsustainable.)

When good people do bad things

To continue my decentring of compassion, or at least of talk of compassion, I want to present an argument that the failures of care that have received such publicity over recent years may not, at least in one sense, be failures of care at all.

After the Stafford scandal and the Francis report, the phrase on the lips of many both outside and inside nursing was 'compassion deficit'. Many said that nursing had lost its way because it had clearly been recruiting the wrong sort, people with good academic qualifications but without 'that caring nature'. What was needed was the more stringent controls on recruitment and selection with which I started the chapter. But it is possible to see these problems not in terms of moral failures but as the effect on cognition (how we perceive and understand what is around us) of certain factors in the context of care delivery – such as being placed under pressure (Paley 2014). We first need to separate two things that are often confused – compassion as an orientation or personal motivation and compassion (or 'helping') as an action. It is quite possible, and indeed in certain circumstances, quite likely, that compassionate people will behave in non-helping ways. A series of experiments undertaken by psychologists show that when conditions are manipulated, people can behave in surprisingly non-helping ways such as stepping over someone (in one example an actor pretending to have a heart attack) who appears to be collapsing on the street. Combined with information about nursing staff shortages at Stafford Hospital, we might conclude that it is not unlikely that 'in these circumstances, attention devoted to one seriously ill patient could prevent the distress of another being recognized' (Paley 2014 p. 6). These experiments suggest the effect of 'inattentional blindness'.

Another set of experiments demonstrates the phenomenon of 'outsider disbelief', much in evidence in response to news reports of NHS failures. In these experiments subjects were asked if they would fail to notice certain apparently obvious events such as the substitution of one person in mid-conversation with an entirely different person while the research subject is momentarily distracted. These experiments consistently showed that indi-viduals' strong disbelief that they could be deceived so easily was not matched by their actual performance.

Social psychologists have extensively investigated the conditions in which people do or do not act in helping ways and found that contextual factors provide a far more powerful explanation than notions of character traits, virtues or compas-sion and that outsiders commonly fail to believe how easily and radically their behaviour and observations can be affected by circumstances. The pages of the Francis reports make no reference to this body of knowledge and perpetuate popular assumptions about caring characteristics and caring work. The final part of this argument draws on experiments such as the 'Stanford Prison' experiment undertaken in 1971, in which college students, with normal personality profiles, were asked to role-play prisoners or prison guards. The experiment ended with the role-playing 'guards' behaving in dehumanizing ways toward the 'prisoners'. After the experiment was stopped the 'guards' were incredulous about their behaviour (Zimbardo 2007). The experimenter concluded that 'social situations can have more profound effects on the behaviour and mental functioning of individuals ... than we might believe possible' (Zimbardo 2007 p. 211). So we could conclude that testing a nurse applicant for the desired values and attitudes before they are placed in particular environments, such as understaffed NHS organizations, will reveal little about how they will behave once they are put in this environment.[8]

Compassion, empathy and alternatives

To summarize my argument so far, nursing has a history of identifying with the strongly subjective concepts of caring, compassion and empathy. The practice of these attributes is said to have therapeutic benefit for patients, is felt to differentiate

8 If I have not made it clear enough already, this argument is John Paley's. It has been critiqued for example by Philip Darbyshire (2014) with a reply by John Paley (2015).

the profession from medicine and forms the basis of what has been called patient-centred care. In a 'post-Francis' managerialist era these very concepts have been used to discipline the profession. Those involved in recruitment are obliged to test for their presence in applicants and researchers have developed instruments to measure whether patients are detecting their incidence in consultations with nurses (Bikker *et al.* 2015). Instead of distancing the profession from this talk, leading UK nurses have tended to reaffirm the profession's identification with caring, compassion and empathy. I am not the first person, however, to think that there may be some unanticipated consequences of nursing's strong identification with this cluster of terms around caring and compassion.[9] I have made the point already that this identification can individualize the way that people inside and outside the profession understand good and bad nursing and distract from a critique of the structure that nurses work within.[10] A little while ago the then general secretary of the RCN spoke at a conference about the value of nursing.[11] His approach was to give examples of when individual nurses had used a mixture of initiative, extra effort and understanding of an act that they felt would be appreciated by a patient. The result was a series of moving stories of empathetic nursing. The problem, however, is that if good nursing can be explained by this personal orientation and special effort on the part of the nurse, then it is a small step to understand examples of poor care in exactly the same terms – we just have not got the right people or they are not trying hard enough. There is also a danger, as many have pointed out, that the skill required to nurse gets overlooked.

9 For a critique of overreliance on the 'virtue script' and its accompanying defocussing on skills see Nelson (1995), and Nelson and Gordon (2006).
10 Such a critique needs to go further than simply repeating the complaint that nurses are too busy to care properly and to include analysis of the effect of aspects of NHS and professional culture, which is what I aim to do with this book.
11 Peter Carter's talk at the RCN Research Society Conference in Glasgow in 2014.

Though not one of the six Cs, largely because it starts with E, many believe that empathy is a vital quality for nurses and even that it forms the essence (another E word) of nursing itself as an ethical (E again) practice (Dinkins 2011). However, as with many ideas in nursing, some of the profession's leaders have overinflated the importance of the concept in order to bolster up the value of nursing work. So empathy has been promoted as an almost religious awareness that nurses have special access to, or as a fuzzy feel-good substitute for thinking.

Perhaps we should look for some definitions of empathy, though we could be forgiven for thinking of the term as an 'empty signifier' where its actual meaning is all but irrelevant and it is the effect of the term that counts.[12] One often paraphrased definition presents empathy as the capacity to understand or feel what another person is experiencing from within that other person's frame of reference, i.e. the capacity to place oneself in another's position (adapted from https://en.wikipedia.org/wiki/Empathy). Histories of the term trace its use from nineteenth-century aesthetics (an observer's feelings that are evoked by gazing at a work of art) through philosophy and psychology to the various twentieth-century thera- peutic occupations. Figures such as Carl Rogers, the founder of 'client centred therapy', emphasized the combination of accurate perception of the client's frame of reference and the separateness of the therapist/observer, perceiving it 'as if' it were one's own (Rogers 1959). So already there are nuanced strands to this concept: a cognitive aspect – an ability to understand the situation of others – and an emotional side – the capacity to feel what others feel. You might want to add two more 'dimensions' to the way that empathy has been described: moral and behavioural (Morse *et al.* 1992). The moral understanding of empathy is

---

12 For example, when I use the term about myself I feel a comforting sense of being part of a special community; the term can stand in for a number of different and possibly unexamined feelings and beliefs about myself and the value of who I am and what I do. When we use it in conversation we can feel a sense of identity, recognition and solidarity because we are using the same word.

highly positively loaded and in the hands of some nurse leaders it is the empathetic work of nurses that elevates them to a status far beyond ordinary occupations. That is a hard calling to live up to for many.[13]

I do think that there are some problems with too strong an identification with empathy, or with emotional empathy on the part of nurses (or any other practitioner aiming to do therapeutic work). Author Leslie Jamison in a debate on empathy in the Boston Review warns:

> It can also offer a dangerous sense of completion: that something has been done because something has been felt. It is tempting to think that feeling someone's pain is necessarily virtuous in its own right.
>
> (Jamison 2014)

Perhaps some nurses stress these qualities to cover over a fear of a lack of knowledge or authority in their practice. It could well be that students tend to emphasize the contribution of empathy and empathetic communication with patients before they come to a full grasp of the skills involved in nursing work, as students themselves in one of my focus groups have suggested. However to look into research writing about empathy in nursing and healthcare we might be surprised by the down to earth and clearly practical way that the concept can be discussed. For example, in an article in the *British Journal of General Practice* on empathy and quality of care (Mercer and Reynolds 2002 p. 9), the authors tell us why empathy might be important in healthcare. This is because it can enable certain things to get done:

> The importance of empathy in the therapeutic relationship is related to the aims of such relationships. Irrespective of

13 Loretta Zderad and Josephine Paterson, two American nurse academics promoted this view, perhaps unintentionally, in a desire to provide nurses with a theory that reflected the relational aspect of nursing work. See their website at http://humanisticnursing.weebly.com/

the context of the therapeutic relationship, there appears to be a core set of common aims or purposes. These include:

1   initiating supportive, interpersonal communication in order to understand the perceptions and needs of the patient;
2   empowering the patient to learn, or cope more effectively with his or her environment; and,
3   reduction or resolution of the patient's problems.

I spoke about putting forward an 'alternative' to empathy at the beginning of this chapter. The writing that I have explored here has already started to set out what this might look like and I will summarize it here. There are a number of problems with a strong belief in empathy, all of them well discussed. First, there is something arrogant or we could say imperialistic about my understanding of you. I can only know you from my own position. At best I have a fantasy of who you are and what you are like. The danger of too strong a belief in the 'common humanity' (Olsen 1991) approach to empathy is the assumption that my experiences and emotional behaviours are the same as yours, that *'I know how you feel'*. For example, your eyes fill with tears when I ask about your mother because you never met her while my eyes fill with tears because I murdered mine and am still angry with her. Second, I do not really know how, or why or what often, *I* feel, at least according to (some forms of) psychoanalysis and their notion of the self divided into conscious and unconscious, the unconscious constantly influencing how I experience the world without my knowing. Third, I may find this prospect of radical aloneness rather too much to bear and seek comfort in fantasies of deep connection and oneness with the humans I come across, for example the patients that I am required to care for. Although there are well-formulated critiques of this line of argument, to entertain the possibility that there may be truth in it makes nursing's talk of empathy start to feel slightly uncomfortable, sinister even if it results in the exploitation of patients for nurses' own emotional needs.

My alternative has already been well articulated by the authors I have looked to in this chapter but I will restate it here. It consists of a combination of constant and careful communication with patients and others in our care, attentive listening and rechecking that we have understood, the adopting of a professional position in relation to them and the ability to have and communicate high levels of knowledge regarding their situation. This is, of course, nothing new but if we arrive at this through a careful critique of the uses and dangers of talk of care, compassion and empathy, and the fuzziness of thought that it can lead to, then we can start to practise as nurses in a more considered and confident way. We might be freed from our anxiety about not being compassionate enough and of being too compassionate.

Chapter 4

Nursing work is difficult work and what to do about it

JACQUELINE (second-year student mental health branch): I initially wanted to do medicine at the beginning – I got good, obviously good grades in biology and stuff and that's what I originally wanted to do but something happened to me at the time so that in a sense acted as a setback to me but then the positive aspect of it was that, you know, the way nurses looked after me then – it was a long time ago – is different compared to now –

Nursing work is difficult for many reasons. Some are unavoidable and some are avoidable. In this chapter I want to discuss some of the results of research into nursing work. Some studies show nursing and healthcare work as stressful: these include psychological studies of burnout as well as ethnographies revealing the subtle and often informal ways that individuals interact with organizations to get the work done, to manage the trauma that is sometimes involved in the work and for other reasons such as to triage patients into those worthy of nursing care and those not. I suggest that many of these ways of interacting and behaving, such as the development of 'front stage' and 'back stage' behaviour, which I will discuss later, can be considered successful from a professional point of view, even though they might initially appear unpalatable.

Here is a list of reasons why nursing might be difficult work. Your challenge is to decide which are the avoidable reasons and which are unavoidable:

dealing with people who are sick and possibly dying;
dealing with these sick people's relatives who might be grateful, worried or angry;
poor relationships with senior colleagues;
feeling that you have too much work to do at the standard you believe it requires;
difficult inter-professional relationships;
lack of respect from managers;
synchronizing family arrangements with working shifts;
feeling conflict between professional values and workplace culture;
insufficient knowledge about patients' conditions;
little decision-making authority in your ward or clinic.

Researchers from different disciplines have studied people at work. Depending on their orientation and their intentions they see different things. 'Time and motion' studies have a long and sometimes derided history. Comedy films from the 1950s show men with white coats and clipboards making notes on factory workers to tell bosses if they are wasting time. Today, this kind of researcher – time and motion I mean not management snitch – will attach GPS devices to nurses on the ward and give them smartphones that vibrate telling them to note down what they are doing at that moment (I am not making this up). Their intention is perhaps not simply to get them to work harder, but to discover how they can be used 'more efficiently', and to re-engineer the hospital to ensure that nurses' work contributes to 'sustainability and affordability of the hospital' (Hendrich et al. 2008). These studies can show that nurses spend a third of their nursing practice on documentation, a fifth on care coordination and nearly the same amount on giving medicines. Nurses can walk between one and five miles during a shift.[1] Such studies can also reveal how fragmented and interrupted nursing work can be (Westbrook *et al.* 2011), especially while giving medicines (National Nursing Research Unit 2010). Alongside these organizational studies, work, and nursing work in particular, has attracted the attention of psychologists who have focussed on and developed a number of related phenomena. I summarize some of these now.

Burnout: a short history

Work psychologists have considered stress as an occupational hazard since the 1950s (Jennings 2008). Many of these studies focus on stress as a predominantly physiological phenomenon – the body's response to an event that threatens its well-being. But more holistic understandings that take into account the personal and social meaning of these so-called 'stressors' are a better place to start. In the mid-1970s American psychologist Herbert Freudenberger coined the term 'burnout' to describe the effects of chronic stress on employees whose work involved continued direct interactions with clients (Freudenberger 1974). He took the term from the illegal drug scene where it was used to refer to the devastating effect of chronic drug abuse. He applied it to the gradual emotional exhaustion, loss of motivation, and reduced commitment among volunteers of the St Mark's Free Clinic, which dealt with drug users in New York, that he observed while working there as a consulting psychiatrist. Freudenberger himself experienced burnout, which, it has been claimed, increased his credibility in spreading the message of burnout (Schaufeli *et al.* 2008).

The investigation of burnout has given the so-called helping professions a new prominence in work psychology as studies, notably those of Christina Maslach, examined the 'frustrated idealism' of many working in the newly expanded human service

---

1   Although the study I am quoting from was done in the United States, these findings will not surprise any nurse working in the UK.

professions in 1960s America. The phenomenon of burnout caught the imagination of the public and the psychology community alike as it revealed a sad reversal of the altruism and optimism of these workers who came to develop negative perceptions and feelings about their clients and patients. Some believe that burnout was in part brought about by a realization by many workers at that time that underlying arrangements in society blocked their efforts to improve the situation of their clients (Schaufeli *et al.* 2008). Maslach described burnout as 'a state of exhaustion in which one is cynical about the value of one's occupation and doubtful of one's capacity to perform' (Maslach *et al.* 1996 p. 20). In times of austerity, assault on welfare and growing societal inequality I leave it to you to decide how far this perception is a distortion or an insight. Perhaps an understanding of these structural factors and an accompanying realistic expectation of the impact of our own work might help us avoid succumbing to this cynicism.

Maslach considered that burnout has three aspects: 'depersonalization' – an attitude of detachment toward clients, 'personal accomplishment' or rather its lack, and 'emotional exhaustion'. She and colleagues developed a questionnaire intended to measure the level of burnout in individuals that has since become widely used around the globe in studies of nurses. The Maslach Burnout Inventory (MBI) has 22 questions scored on a scale from 1 'Never' to 6 'Every Day'. Scores above certain points on each of the three aspects named above are considered to indicate levels of burnout. How much burnout is there among nurses? Different studies claim to have detected widely different levels. One recent large study of hospital nurses carried out in 12 countries in Europe (Sermeus *et al.* 2011) found burnout varied from 44% of nurses in Greece, via 42% of nurses in England to only 4.2% in Germany. Studies point to various causes of burnout: excessive workload, long shifts and shiftwork, dealing with sickness and death, role ambiguity and poor relationships with managers. Personal factors such as age and marital status have also been claimed to influence levels of burnout. Unsurprisingly many have offered advice about avoiding burnout. As we noted in our discussion in Chapter 2 of how resilience has been promoted, this advice tends to feature personal strategies sometimes accompanied with pessimism about the possibility of positive change in the NHS workplace. For example, one writer in a helpful review recommends individual reflection as a more realistic option compared with clinical supervision because the promise of clinical supervision that is then thwarted because of workplace failures to prioritize it can actually do more harm than good (Fearon and Nicol 2011).

Emotional labour

'Emotional labour' is sometimes discussed alongside burnout as a common problematic feature of nursing work. Let's look at where the term came from and its original meaning because it is easy to misunderstand it – and in any case it applies in a more complicated way to health service work than it does to service sector private corporations to whose work it was first applied.[2]

What about this provocative definition: emotional labour describes the commodification of workers' emotions and their alienation from their own feelings in the workplace? When employers train their workers to smile at clients and show a concern for them through a range of physical gestures with the expectation that those clients will find that service pleasing and return, that is emotional labour. Emotional labour will involve both expressing a certain range of acceptable emotions and not expressing other unacceptable emotions. Acceptable emotions in most jobs would be welcome, warmth, energy, empathy and interest in the client. Unacceptable emotions would include disinterest, disapproval, impatience and disgust. Debt collectors,

2   Generally it is the American sociologist Arlie Hochschild who is credited with inventing the term and putting it into the vocabulary of the sociology of work. She proposed that in any social situation particular emotions come to be considered appropriate. Her seminal work, *The Managed Heart*, included examples of emotional labour in the work of flight attendants Hochschild (1983).

on the other hand, as has been pointed out, are trained in ways of expressing impatience. Researchers have differentiated between surface and deep acting as strategies that employees use to regulate these emotions. 'Surface acting' is considered to be the broadly conscious 'faking' of emotions that the workers know they are not feeling. 'Deep acting' is a more subtle idea. Here workers make efforts to connect with and express some genuine emotions. This might involve something like the way that 'method' actors conjure up personal memories in order to think themselves into a part.[3] However, aspects of professional training, for example those that teach about how fear might cause patients or carers to behave in an angry way, can make shifts in how nurses or doctors feel and respond when confronted with such behaviour. Added to this, empathy is such a strong feature of professional socialization in nursing that it provides a resource or a shared feeling rule, to use a term from the emotional labour literature,[4] that nurses can draw on. Or to put it another way, nurses identify with the caring role required of a nurse. This might make acting in an empathetic way easier and less jarring though, as I suggested in earlier chapters, it can have its own hazards. Research generally shows that workers who predominantly engage in 'deep acting' experience less long-term stress than their surface acting colleagues (Grandey 2003).

Emotional labour might also include the suppression of the emotions of employees that could, in other situations, be considered positive, such as a desire to be honest felt by a flight attendant needing to communicate calmly to passengers in a crisis situation. It is not difficult to imagine a nurse in a similar predicament. I will talk about this later.

But what kind of emotional labour is required in nursing? By comparing nursing work with the emotional work expected

3   Method actors include Johnny Depp, Anne Hathaway and Christian Bale.
4   Some writers argue that the term 'display rules' is a more accurate term because it is the emotions that ought to be publicly expressed rather than what emotions are actually felt which is at stake (Ashforth and Humphrey 1993).

of a waitress we can perhaps identify some of the key features of nursing work. One researcher describes in detail her job as a waitress in a high-end restaurant (Dowling 2007). The restaurant had produced a booklet *Philosophy of Hospitality* used for training its staff and orientating them to how they were expected to behave – in line with company policy certainly but expected to 'use' their own personality and individuality.

> We are throwing a party – it's going to be very hip and fun, lots of people will be coming and going. We want our guests to feel at home and cared for. We have to make them feel that they are the only ones at the party that are important to us. We never want our guests to feel ignored, unwelcome or rushed. You are the key . . . you have to be the perfect host or hostess: cheery, relaxed, unflappable. You set the tone for each table the way you greet each guest. In short, you are graceful, sincere and refined. We will achieve this by anticipating guest needs.
>
> (p. 120)

As the author, Emma Dowling, a PhD student when she wrote this, points out, it is the desire for profit – capital – that drives this concern with the diner's experience and the philosophy is, as she says, imposed by management.[5] Waiters and waitresses in this restaurant are given detailed instruction about when to smile and greet guests but crucially are expected to draw on their own natural abilities to achieve the desired customer experience and act out the 'core values' of the establishment.

5   Who are the 'managers'? Emma Dowling writes: 'I use "management" as a shorthand for the structure which acts on behalf of and in the interest of capital' (Dowling 2007 p. 119). It could be argued that today's NHS managers, through close scrutiny of financial expenditure coupled with the requirement to give an account for the meeting of targets e.g. throughput – required quality indicators – are placed into a position where their work is closely similar to the work of managers who work in for-profit corporations.

Try reading the passage above from the *Philosophy* and replace 'guest' with 'patient', 'host' and 'hostess' with 'nurse', 'table' with 'bay' and 'hip' with 'hip-replacement' (not really). Could this be a philosophy from your trust? 'We are throwing a party': what could be the NHS or nursing equivalent?

In this restaurant there are weekly incentives – prizes for the employee who is considered to have best exemplified the core values but there are also slightly more sinister motivators in the form of 'the mystery diner'. A mystery diner is commonplace in the service industry. Restaurants engage mystery dining firms to assess how well the dining experience meets the standards set by management. TV comedies, including *Fawlty Towers* which focuses on an inept guesthouse manager, present these mystery figures as opportunities for farce; however, what is perhaps surprising is that in the real world such agents record minute details about the time taken by the waitress to first approach the table, what time they take the order for food, how much time passed before the drinks arrived and every aspect of her performance throughout the entire meal. Such information would be collated and compared with other parts of the restaurant and previous visit performance. These figures would be used by managers as incentives for staff or as opportunities for extra training.[6]

So there are some apparent similarities between emotional labour in the hospitality industry and healthcare. But the comparison highlights what makes nursing unusual and unusually

6   Does this sound familiar? See the Care Quality Commission (CQC) website www.cqc.org.uk/content/what-we-do-inspection for a description of the NHS and social care mystery diner.

demanding work.[7] Although a meal out can go badly wrong, you would have to be unlucky in your choice of restaurant to encounter fear, suffering and death at the dinner table. But at least one of these three, if not all, can be a central feature of the work of a nurse. Because of this the emotional labour of the nurse is likely to be different from that of a waitress or flight attendant. At a simple level, which is easy to take for granted, nurses are expected to respond to patients 'professionally', with an interested but detached, unflappable, confidence-inspiring demeanour, with a clear inflection of kindness. In this context display rules discourage the exhibition of fear, grief and disgust, as well perhaps of more organizationally induced emotions of tiredness, frustration, boredom or anger.

Some accounts of emotional labour in nursing leave out the part played by capital – or rather by a management that sees it as part of its role to 'manage' the emotional displays of its workers to its own benefit. Leaving out this essential feature of emotional labour as conceived by Hochschild, leaves you with the rather less politically engaged observation that nursing work is emotionally demanding because nurses experience emotions that they do not express with patients and sometimes co-workers. So where, in nursing, is the equivalent of the management training for new waiters and waitresses, the *Philosophy of Hospitality* handbook and the mystery diner reporting on the performance of the nurse? Attempts to manage the emotion work of nurses are on the rise. First there are attempts at 'values based recruitment' to the profession (see Chapter 3) to select only those who show themselves to be compassionate and non-judgemental. Then there are an increasing number of documents and policies seeking to ensure that nurses display the six Cs, for example the Care in Practice project (Commissioning Board Chief Nursing Officer 2012). Finally there are the relatively new

---

7   Among the first writers to take the notion of emotional labour into studies of nursing were Nicky James (1989) and Pam Smith (1992).

scrutinies from government agencies and independent regulators. See the Care Quality Commission's description of how the NHS and Social care mystery diner can make scheduled and unscheduled visits asking patients whether they were treated with care and understanding by staff.[8] We might call these managerial attempts to shape the display rules that nurses are expected to pay attention to. But there is another, deeper set of display rules at work. The profession has a much longer identification with altruistic and caring values than the UK NHS's recent wake up after the events at Stafford and elsewhere as I have shown in the previous chapter. In fact it is this deep identification with caring that makes working in today's NHS so jarring an experience for many clinicians. They feel that it is managerial processes, shortages of staff and lack of time that thwart their desire to *be* caring. Nurses are ambivalent about initiatives like the six Cs and the Care in Practice project. On the one hand they support something that restates their own values. On the other they see reorganizations, endless attempts to contain costs and set performance targets as preventing them from acting out those values to their own satisfaction. So this is another aspect of emotional labour in nursing – deep ambiguity about the display rules at work. One set of rules requires caring and compassion while another says 'act like you have care and compassion but above all keep up with the pace of work'. It is to this fundamental dilemma that I will now turn.

Nursing work in depth

The kind of research I have talked about at the start of this chapter can give us a flavour of nursing work but ethnographic studies, where researchers observe in a far more open-ended way and, to a certain extent, actually participate in nursing work,

8   See www.cqc.org.uk/content/what-we-do-inspection. The question about treatment by staff with care and understanding is one of many included by the CQC in its surveys of NHS performance.

can tell us a far more nuanced story of what is important to nurses themselves, and how they explain what they do. Thankfully nursing is not short of this kind of work, most of it done by nurses themselves for PhD studies, but some done by 'outsiders'. One of my favourites, which started as a PhD by an 'outsider' is Daniel Chambliss' careful ethnographic work on ethical decision-making and socialization (Chambliss 1996) among nurses. Although it was carried out in US hospitals in the 1980s and 1990s his work still reads as highly relevant for nurses in today's NHS. Although our word 'resilience' does not appear once in his index, the whole book, in a way, is a description of resilience in action. And it is very different from the version of individual elasticity that we discussed earlier in this book. He sees that the whole hospital setting (his work was done in hospitals) and particularly routines, both official and unofficial, enable nurses to continue to function in highly pressured and often traumatic situations.

First he focuses on what might be called desensitization (he uses the term 'flattening of emotion' p. 12), a phenomenon that is often considered negative and even dangerous – it has been offered as one explanation of the events at Stafford Hospital. His conclusion from interviews with more than 100 nurses over 15 years and a total of 2 years' fieldwork is that in order to work effectively in the healthcare environment, workers have to routinize the traumatic. Part of this routinization involves the sharing of 'back stage' (Goffman 1959) humour about horrific situations and events and apparently disparaging labelling of certain classes of patients. (See Chapter 9 on social media for examples of nurses and doctors confusing the front and back stages – never a good idea.) The strength of Chambliss' work is that he does not make moral judgements about this aspect of socialization. Instead he understands the function that it serves within healthcare work. The layperson walking into any busy trauma unit, for example, would be unable to help and not just because of a lack of skill. To illustrate his point about the routinization of trauma he describes from his field notes the inhabitants of the eight rooms in the surgical intensive care unit one Saturday evening and how nurses view them:

Room 1. 64-year-old white woman with an aortic valve replacement; five separate IMEDs [intravenous drop-control devices] feeding in nitroglycerine, vasopressors, Versed [a pain killer which also blocks memory]. Foley [catheter in the bladder], a pulse oximeter on her finger, a[rterial monitoring] line. Diabetic. In one 30-second period during the night, her blood pressure dropped from 160/72 to 95/50, then to 53/36, before the nurse was able to control the drop. Nurses consider her 'basically healthy'.

(Chambliss 1996 p. 17)

Alongside routinization, the other key ingredient that makes nursing special, he says, is the dilemma that nurses experience regarding conflicting demands. On the one hand they lack formal organizational authority – the power exercised by doctors and administrators – and on the other they have a strong professional ethic. Chambliss tells us that day-to-day nursing is all about coping with this dilemma:

The nurse is a paid employee of the hospital,[9] but she is more than that. She is actively encouraged to be, simultaneously, a caring person, a committed professional, and a loyal subordinate. Obviously, these components of her role frequently conflict with each other.

(p. 180)

The stories told in Chambliss' book, many of them gruesome, show nurses acting out resilience. The 'checklists' of resilience that we saw in Chapters 1 and 2 include the advice to 'have a sense of humour'. Chambliss' ethnography shows that nurses certainly have a sense of humour but often the humour is

---

9   Nurses working in the UK may be employed by a private company, but it is more likely that they work within the country's National Health Service. This provides another layer of complexity. The NHS is an idealistic symbol toward which employees and many users feel great affection and loyalty. But it is also constantly reorganized by governments and the object of periodic fierce financial cutbacks. It is the solution but also the problem.

completely unpalatable in anything other than the most private of professional settings and forged out of the most extreme human horror. Their jokes would never make it onto resilience websites. Their humour is nevertheless a creative response to almost impossible situations featuring human tragedy, indifferent doctors and organizational subjection.

What might resilience mean? Supervision and peer-support

So, in the light of all this, what might resilience mean for nurses? As I have said before, understanding how situations came to exist gives us power. Nursing the sick is going to be difficult work, but the conditions under which it is done can make it even more difficult. Being able to untangle the political and organizational causes (your manager is in danger of reprimand for not meeting a unit target and puts you under pressure to speed up discharge) from the direct human causes (your patient requires CPR because they have stopped breathing) and to trace how each situation came to be as well as how they interact can help develop resilience. Being more conscious about the fact that you are engaged in emotional labour can do the same.

Consciousness-raising is better with others. Supervision, formal or informal and peer-support, again either formally arranged or more informal, can help build bonds and aid understanding of the pressures and decisions made 'up stream' that affect your day-to-day working life. Ground rules for these groups or meetings could include:

Making the effort to be analytical rather than complaining,
Focussing on structures and processes rather than individuals, and
Being non-judgemental about our own behaviour.

What about starting from a particular event, either something that went well or something that didn't, and working backwards, perhaps all the way to general government policy?

(See the end of Chapter 2 for more ideas about working in groups to increase resilience.)

Chapter 5

Nursing: whose idea was it anyway?

PENNY (Postgraduate Diploma second-year student): I think the NHS depends a lot on good faith and they like to use, like sort of emotional blackmail. This is my experience because I've worked in the NHS for 20-odd years [in laboratories before nurse training]. It's kind of like, well you shouldn't be complaining because, you know, there's sick people and they need the money, rather than like refurbish your tea room. The patients need the money but then in reality it doesn't really work that way because the money never comes to the patients. It's just like in this mythical ether somewhere. (laughter)

MICHAEL: So what were you saying, you said emotional blackmail?

PENNY: Yeah I think the whole sort of 'oh it's sick people' and you can't expect to have a certain standard of facilities and what not. You know what I mean?

MICHAEL: So how does that message get around?

PENNY: It's just a general consensus I think, it's a culture of martyrdom (laughs)

OTHERS: Martyrs! Martyrs! (laughter)

Understanding how we got here means looking at where we came from. The word 'evolution' has been used to describe how nursing has changed from its nineteenth-century roots to the present day.[1] This metaphorical

---

1   This is most noticeable in texts about nursing by US authors starting from the beginning of the twentieth century but intensifying from the 1980s. If you are interested, take the briefest of glimpses at: (Meleis 1985; Nutting and Dock 1907).

use of the biological concept carries with it ideas of development and progress underpinned by continuity all pushed forward by some kind of morally positive unseen hand. Instead of this view I want, in this chapter, to set out a brief background to contemporary nursing that shows how different groups have struggled for power not only over how the profession is organized but also over how it is understood and viewed – over what nursing *is*. My journey through this history will be mainly chronological but sometimes thematic.

At last – an occupation for respectable women

What we know as nursing in the UK and in many other countries of the world was invented in mid-nineteenth-century Britain. Before that we can trace religious orders of both men and women whose work included caring for the sick. After their decline, a more informal and usually derided assortment of women offered an array of services to the sick where they lived. The treatment of illness was home-based before the rise of hospitals toward the end of the nineteenth century. Florence Nightingale (1820–1910) is described as a reformer because her project was to take the discredited persona and activity of these individuals and refashion them into an occupation that could be considered on the right side of respectability to attract educated women. Like many figures with a political mission she painted an exaggerated picture of what she was up against, writing that nursing had been left to 'those who were too old, too weak, too drunken, too dirty, too stupid or too bad to do anything else' (Gaffney 1982 p. 139). Nightingale's project was aided by the rise of medicine with the discovery of anaesthetics and antiseptic surgery as well as the success of the medical profession itself. This created a need for a worker like a nurse to staff an increasing number of hospital wards.[2]

2　Another major driver was Nightingale's publicizing of poor nursing care provided to British soldiers in the Crimean War that led to the establishment of military hospitals and the recruitment of nurses to them.

Nightingale faced two challenges: to make the often intimate physical work of nursing acceptable to respectable women and to make the employment of such women acceptable to highly patriarchal Victorian society that generally viewed women's role as exclusively to do with homemaking and child-rearing.[3] A solution to both was to conceive of nursing and especially nurse training as a highly disciplined moral as well as technical training and to emphasize nurses' subservience to medical practitioners rather than their possible rivalry in the professional arena. So while nursing represented a new opportunity for female employment and education it also embodied sharp divisions in role and status in the workplace, notably between male doctors and female nurses.

Are we better off like doctors or not?

Very soon there were conflicting ideas about what nursing was and could be. The spectacular success of medicine at laying a claim to a field of work, keeping everyone else out, and at achieving social status and financial reward not surprisingly attracted some early nurse leaders. They believed that adopting the tactics of doctors was the way to establish the profession. The Medical Act had been passed by parliament in 1858. It set up the General Medical Council and instigated the medical register, a public list of all medical practitioners. Medicine had convinced the government that it had a body of knowledge of unique social value and medicine took an ever greater role in public life. But nursing was divided on whether to push for state registration and the form that it should take. As a result the various bills promoted by nursing and other organizations and individuals in parliament all failed to be passed and it was not until after the First World War that a bill devised by the government eventually (1919) became law and the nursing register opened.

3   Married women could not 'engage in trade'. (Women were not admitted into the top universities until well into the twentieth century in some cases).

The registration of nurses promised a standard and state-recognized training and qualification for nurses. Symbolically it marked the achievement of professional status.

Nursing after the Second World War

After the battering of World War Two (1939–45), Britain faced the challenge of rebuilding a peacetime economy and many workers were in short supply. The newly formed National Health Service (1948) also required staff. The solution was to encourage mass migration. Various schemes enabled young German women to come to Britain to work in the cotton industry in the north of the country but also to work as nurses (Weber-Newth and Steinert 2006). The most well-discussed recruitment and resulting migration, however, was from the British Colonies, in particular the West Indies. The website historyandpolicy.org describes how the Ministries of Labour and of Health along with the Colonial Office and nursing organizations set out to recruit hospital staff from the Caribbean. They focussed on auxiliary workers, nurses and students as well as domestics. The colonies and former colonies supplied Britain with cheap labour that met NHS staffing shortages for many decades. By the mid-1960s, 3–5,000 Jamaican nurses were working in British hospitals and by the early 1970s approximately 10,500 students had been recruited from overseas. However, the recruitment left a shameful legacy in terms of racism and discrimination. Many nurses who arrived in the UK from the Caribbean during the 1950s expected to be studying for the State Registered Nurse qualification (the predecessor to the present RGN – Registered General Nurse) and intended to return home to gain employment as a nurse. However, nursing bodies at the time argued that these students' racial characteristics limited their intellectual capabilities and motivation:

> Many overseas nurses were forced or even duped into State Enrolled Nurse (SEN) training rather than the more prestigious and more highly valued SRN qualification. The longer term consequences of this were significant as the SEN was

not an internationally-recognized qualification and limited overseas nurses' options for returning home.

(Snow and Jones 2011)

Today black nurses are still likely to experience racism in the NHS from some patients and in terms of career development (Allan *et al.* 2009).

'We need to do something about nursing': modernizing and more

Although nursing has rarely occupied the policy limelight, culturally the profession has remained close to the British public's heart. The media have projected fantasies onto nurses that have to varying degrees been enjoyed by the public. The more well-known stereotypes are of the highly sexualized woman and of the angelic helper and healer (Hallam 2000, Fealy 2004), reflecting perhaps general stereotypes applied to women. More complex is the Lady Macbeth nurse whose cruelty is all the more shocking because it is seen as an abomination to her sex.[4] In fiction she appears in films such as Miloš Forman's *One Flew Over the Cuckoo's Nest* (1975) in the form of the apparently frustrated and sadistic Nurse Ratched employed in an unenlightened mental institution and, arguably, in Anthony Minghella's beautifully photographed *The English Patient* (1996), where nurse Hana played by Juliette Binoche kills Ralph Fiennes with a morphine overdose in a consensual act of mercy killing that the NMC would urge real nurses not to emulate. In the realm of fact she takes the form of nurses who have murdered their patients and shocked the country, one such nurse, in the 1990s being referred to as 'the angel of death' (Batty 2007). And if, by any chance, the wrongdoer is a migrant nurse, the racist press

---

4   Shakespeare's Lady Macbeth calls on the spirits to 'unsex' her and tells Macbeth that she would be prepared to pluck her nipple from the boneless gums of a smiling baby she is feeding and dash its brains out (Act 1, Scene 7). And we thought Hilary Clinton was hard core.

is keen to point this out to make sure the population is constantly on its guard against dangers from beyond its borders.[5]

In the less dramatic world of policy, the training of nurses staggered into the higher education sector in the early to mid-1990s, 20 years after a government report had called for a thorough reform of nursing and midwifery regulation and education.[6] There was a sense that 'we need to do something about nursing'. Before the all-seeing NMC, nurses, midwives, health visitors and others were regulated by a body with a much longer name. The publishers have asked me not to name it here as it will use up too much ink. This body, with considerable consultation and help from outside the profession, devised what it rather timidly called Project 2000 whereby nurses would be taught in higher education institutions rather than on site in the health service. Bit by bit those who teach nurses packed up their desks and left hospital schools of nursing and moved into Polytechnic offices, brand new if they were lucky. Then almost before nurse tutors had unpacked their last text book onto Polytechnic bookshelves, the Polys, the once vocationally orientated poor sister to traditional universities, were turned, by the 1992 Further and Higher Education Act into proper universities too. And nurses in training became university students. Surprisingly, the profession seemed to want it. Even nurse managers understood that the increasingly complex work of the nurse required a more highly educated worker, while the

---

5   See some of the coverage of Filipino nurse Victorino Chua who was convicted of murdering patients at Stepping Hill hospital in Manchester. After detailing his crimes, an article in the Daily Mail warns readers: 'NHS chiefs are still hiring nurses from the Philippines, despite the scandal of Victorino Chua, the Mail can reveal today'. www.dailymail.co.uk/news/article-3088513/Did-Filipino-nurse-murder-11-Coroner-reveals-planning-inquests-suspicious-deaths-Stepping-Hill-NHS-poisoner-jailed-35-years.html#ixzz4G4onB6Np

6   If you are really curious this was the Briggs Report. The Briggs in question was historian Asa Briggs. As a report published in 1972 we can consider it history and consign it, in this book, to the footnotes.

architects of the scheme realized that they needed to attract more bright school leavers into the profession, and they were unlikely to be impressed by nursing's old-fashioned and untransferable apprentice-like training scheme. Student nurses were turned, by the magic wand of legislation, from slavish extra pairs of hands useful for making beds into supernumerary participant observers, to borrow a term from anthropologists. At the same time as this professional triumph, the government of the day started to get more interested than ever in the employment of people – health care assistants – who could help these new more educated and likely more expensive nurses.

Reactionary voices, also, were whispering that all this learning was getting in the way of those classic female qualities of common sense, practicality and niceness. And some politicians probably agreed. (Some nurses probably secretly agreed.) If only our nurses could be a little more stupid then everything would be alright again. And those grand universities are surely putting off the armies of nice but slightly dim women who would make *ideal* nurses. But that was then. Today we have all-degree entry into the profession and things are completely different. People are saying 'If only our nurses could be a little more stupid then everything would be alright again, and those grand universities . . .'

But government health policy, particularly during the early years of Tony Blair's 'New Labour' leadership (from 1997), took nursing at its word, passed legislation and made changes to the workings of the NHS that put nurses in prominent and, in theory, responsible positions: Modern Matrons, Nurse Consultants, the nurse-led NHS Direct and even the encouragement, for a while, of Nurse Entrepreneurs. In 2000 the Chief Nursing Officer published 'Ten key roles for nurses', reflecting areas of work that had been promoted by earlier legislation (Department of Health 2000), some of them previously the realm of doctors. See Chapter 6 for more detail. Things were starting to look good. Then we had the recession. Then we had the Conservative-Liberal coalition. Then we had 'austerity'.

Fallen angels?

Nurses cost money to employ and money to train. The Prime Minister's Commission on nursing and midwifery (Prime Minister's Commission 2010) identified that in the year 2008–2009 pre-registration education and support for those professions cost nearly £1 billion: around £568 million for tuition costs and over £352 million for bursaries. (No wonder the government is keen to lose bursary costs.) Recruitment of nurses depends largely on the numbers being trained. In times of austerity governments look to the public sector to find savings. Because the cost of providing nursing care forms such a large part of healthcare costs we tend to get what has been called a 'boom or bust' approach to the number of nurses trained (Buchan 1993, Buchan 2013). The number contracts as managers are forced to reduce costs in times of pressure. Then when the resulting shortages of qualified nurses become apparent in the service, NHS organizations are forced to send teams to journey overseas on recruitment drives and at the same time to engage the far more costly agency nursing staff. But now the challenge for those who are generously called workforce planners is more complicated.

Running the health service is like hugging a balloon. Squeeze in here and something bulges out somewhere else. Once the significant cost to the NHS of employing agency workers, including nurses and doctors, was publicized, Monitor (the sector regulator for health services in England particularly for Foundation trusts) and the NHS Trust Development Authority (which supports non-foundation trusts) started to set expenditure limits on agency spending (Dunn 2016). This started in 2015 and the limits were gradually tightened with elaborate reporting requirements and denial of access to certain funding sources for any trust that exceeded the limits in emergency situations. But one problem was much more difficult to solve. And that problem can be encapsulated in one word – Stafford. The failures of care at Stafford General Hospital, discussed at more length in Chapter 3, showed, in a sense, the logical conclusion of an NHS that strongly incentivizes its managers to contain costs.

So now managers and planners are expected, while maintaining normal service, to control: overall staff costs, agency staff costs and ensure adequate levels of patient safety along with the compassion and 'values' of their staff. The point I am getting to, which is the heading of this section, is that the highly publicized failures of nursing at Stafford and in other places tarnished the generally angelic and trustworthy image that nursing had with the public. In public discussion concern over nurses' moral identity has often seemed to eclipse their technical effectiveness and skill. The events at Stafford emboldened those, mentioned above, who blamed it all on nurses going to university. However, an awareness of the potential dangers of inadequate nursing staffing levels seems to have emerged as a positive, but still tentative, outcome of the Francis report into Stafford, with the release, for example, of guidance on 'Hard Truths commitments regarding the publishing of staffing data' issued in early 2014 (Chief Nursing Officer for England and National Quality Board 2014).

What's next? Nurses in debt and another new worker

Two new pieces of government planning present an opportunity for critique. We are assured that the timing of the proposal for the instigation of a new grade of healthcare worker and the announcement of the scrapping of the bursary for new nursing and other healthcare students from 2017 are merely coincidental. But let's see if the two are linked in any ideological way.

In 2016 Health Education England (HEE) opened a consultation on their plan to develop a new health and social care role. They called it a 'nursing associate' and said that it would be created for a skill level somewhere between existing Healthcare Support Workers and registered nurses.[7] HEE claims the benefits could be increased local workforce capacity i.e. managers

---

7   The proposal was one of 34 recommendations from the Raising the Bar report (Willis 2015).

will be able to afford to engage more staff having perhaps a bigger pool to draw from, and the creation of an additional route into registered nursing for those for whom traditional nurse education (that is soon going to leave students with £50,000 debt – see below) is not feasible. The creation of support grade workers has not been unusual in the public sector in recent years. It is a response to the reduction of budgets that has become not only 'common sense' but seen by managers as an opportunity to think afresh about how to organize healthcare at a local level. However, those planning to introduce supporting/lower paid/ quicker to train/more flexible workers into any setting need to reassure established professionals that the advantages of the new role outweigh the threats. A common approach is to emphasize that the existence of the support role can raise the status of the remaining professionals because they will become concentrated on valuable, technically complex or 'core' work (i.e. work befitting a proper professional). The reality may be, however, that their work becomes increasingly managerial and administrative. One professional fear is that the existence of new assistant-grade workers reduces demand for professionals and threatens their status if lesser-trained workers are able to take on aspects of their work. Those promoting new roles typically emphasize limits and accountability processes to try to counter fears about the safety of the workers. A pattern in nursing education and professionalism is that increases in educational status of the registered nurse are followed shortly after by increased attention to skill mix in the service. It is worth mentioning that the proposal comes at a time when research into mortality in hospitals and its association with the levels of qualified nurses required per patient are circulating (Griffiths *et al.* 2016).

In terms of political ideology (see next chapter) at a broad level the proposal represents a managerialist view of work that sees traditional professional boundaries as a barrier to efficient and flexible working. Traditionally, professions have sought to put boundaries around their work that can only be crossed by those with credentials provided by the profession itself (Witz 1990). Developing a range of ways that those outside the profession can enter, while good from the point of view of equality of opportunity, might be seen by the profession as encroachments on its status and self-determination. So this move can be understood as an example of a common State-profession conflict. How it will play out will depend on the details. By the time you read this, the proposal is likely to have been implemented.

In December 2015 the English Department of Health released a policy paper. This is its summary:

> From 1 August 2017, new nursing, midwifery and allied health students will no longer receive NHS bursaries. Instead, they will have access to the same student loans system as other students.
>
> We intend that students studying nursing, midwifery and the allied health subjects as a second degree will also be able to get student loans.
>
> The change will only affect new students starting their courses from 1 August 2017.
>
> We plan to run a consultation in early 2016 to ask how we can successfully deliver the reforms.
>
> (Department of Health 2015)

As already mentioned, clearly the advantage of this new approach to the DoH is that it can, at a stroke, save at least £500M from its budget.[8] The announcement also brings nursing and allied health professions students into line with medical students who already take out student loans. The Department, and those who support the change, say that this will take an artificial restriction from supply for nursing places because currently the body that commissions nurse education is limited in its number of places and nursing courses are highly

---

8 This potential saving has been questioned by a study commissioned by the unions UNISON and NUS. This study suggests that the change will lead to a fall in recruitment causing an increase in agency spending (Conlon and Ladher 2016).

oversubscribed. What is the ideology here? As I have mentioned elsewhere in this book, the neoliberalism that has been dominating world politics for at least the last 30 years is strongly individualist in character. More collectivist politics tends to see education as a state responsibility because a better educated population is an advantage for all, culturally, politically and economically. Education can also serve to bring equality to society if it is properly available to all regardless of ability to access it and that can bring social cohesion. This is the principle behind government grants for education that still provide free university education in many other countries. For the neoliberal, society is made up of individuals, each with the ability to maximize their own utility through the choices they make, to continually improve their own economic and personal situation. They will be motivated both by what can be achieved and by witnessing those who fail. It is this motivation that leads to invention, innovation, efficiency and, ultimately, wealth. The role of the State from this point of view is not to do anything to get in the way of this free market of individuals. Higher education can be turned into a market to enable this to happen. Universities can be set to compete against each other for market share – that's students. Students can be persuaded to invest in their own future by paying for access to university courses. Their incentive is, hopefully, the better standard of living that a university qualification may give them in the future, although the UK has a high proportion of overqualified workers. Because few people can afford to pay the £9,000 per year that a university degree currently costs, the government have created a mechanism for loans via the Student Loans Company originally set up in 1990, to facilitate the proper operation of the education market. In addition the rate of interest charged to students has been increased to a current maximum of 3.9%. This means that some students are accumulating interest by as much as £180 each month (Collinson 2016).

As with the 'associate nurse' proposal the nursing profession is divided in its view on this initiative, and this largely reflects the interests that different nursing organizations and groups have. The Council of Deans (CoD) is the organization that represents the heads of UK university health faculties providing education for nursing, midwifery and the allied health professions. The CoD argues for the changes because it believes that it will allow the NHS to be more flexible in the number of nurses it employs as it expects the changes to create a larger pool of students to draw from on the familiar grounds that currently nursing courses are highly oversubscribed. CoD also takes pains to point out that students will be financially better off during their course with a student loan than with the current bursary system. Universities may see a financial advantage to this change as the existing 'tariff', the amount that education commissioners pay universities per student, barely covers costs.

The Royal College of Nursing and UNISON on the other hand are against the proposal arguing that it is likely to deter students from poorer backgrounds who do not want to accumulate debt. Because of this the change threatens to reduce the number of nurses in training and hence reduce the size of the future nursing workforce. It has been suggested that students could end their course with up to £65,000 of debt to repay. Currently students start to repay this loan when they earn around £21,000 per year so the repayments would apply to Band 5 nurses. It has been estimated that they would repay approximately £5.25 per month from their salary. This does not take account of interest that still accrues when those with the loan are not earning sufficient to start repayments.

Student groups, such as the National Union of Students (NUS), are also against this move and have campaigned strongly against it. Many argue that they would not have taken up nursing under such conditions and that future generations, particularly from poorer backgrounds will also be discouraged from considering the profession.

Where are we now?

Nursing's history has left a legacy. Despite the successes first of registration, and then of university education, many in the public, many politicians and many nurses want nurses to be nice rather than clever – or nice first and clever when it is absolutely necessary. We can learn from this very brief look at nursing's history that this large and diverse occupation is often divided on the big issues that it has to deal with. Some of this discord reflects the different interests at work across the profession. All of this history is embedded and subtly at work in day-to-day actions in the world of healthcare. To be critical we need to understand all this. As we have seen, the profession unavoidably interacts with the world of national politics so now it is time to turn to the world of politicians.

Chapter 6

Politicians: part of the solution and part of the problem

KEVIN (second-year student mental health branch): But yeah, it's interesting that people are motivated by wanting to see changes – I kind of seesaw backwards and forwards between thinking I don't want to be part of this [profession], this is not, you know, what I signed up for really and thinking, actually, I want to get in there and get a very senior position where I can make things different. You know, it's kind of, so I kind of seesaw a little bit with that.

In this chapter I want to introduce a little of the theory of how national policy is made, discussing influences on the process such as the role of the media, politicians' perceived need for the quick-fix solution, the role of the scientific community and of ideology. I will dwell a little on neoliberalism because many see it as the dominant force in politics today. I will ask what is democracy and is it any good? I will give some examples of politics in action, the welfare state, nurses as the policy instruments of politicians and the healthcare quasi-market. Finally I will make some suggestions about what nurses can do.

Are politicians to be trusted?

Trust in politicians in the UK is low. Social Research company Ipsos MORI says:

> at no point since 1983 have more than a quarter of the public ever trusted politicians to tell the truth. The lowest trust score was recorded in 2009 in the wake of the expenses scandal

[among members of parliament], when only 13% said they trusted politicians.

(Ipsos MORI 2016)

And in mid-2016, after the UK referendum on leaving or remaining in the European Union, the exposure of obvious deceptions particularly from those campaigning for leaving and the failure of those responsible for calling the referendum or campaigning for leaving to take responsibility for the result, many are outraged that politicians' behaviour has slumped to a new low. As a member of one of the major healthcare professions you could also be forgiven for thinking that politicians have little respect for professional views and values. They impose costly and disruptive changes on the system as a whole based on little evidence, embark on macho confrontations with junior doctors (Simms 2016), dispense with nursing policy advice at the Department of Health (Bhardwa 2016) and remove bursary funding for student nurses forcing those who want to enter the profession to take on significant personal debt (Gill 2016). There are countless examples of political actions that appear, at least, to be focussed on making the work of nurses and other healthcare and public sector workers as difficult as possible.

In April 2010, Andrew Lansley, soon to be health secretary in the new Conservative-Liberal coalition, addressed the RCN Congress in the run up to the general election that saw his party elected. His main theme was that NHS staff know best how to run the service and that he would make sure that the NHS has autonomy to ensure there is 'no political interference day by day'. He also said that NHS budget would be 'protected and increasing'. Weeks later and once in office he launched one of the most unpopular and disruptive changes to the structure of the NHS for little tangible benefit. The changes gave rise to almost universal condemnation from doctors, nurses and other groups working in the service yet, with some compromises, were forced through. What is the logic I am proposing is in effect here? That politics involves saying in public what is palatable in order to win support while keeping actual policy intentions hidden. Here is one of many possible examples of why trust in politicians is low.

In this chapter I want to try to discover the logic that operates in the UK's political system. If we are to be critically resilient we cannot afford to be ill informed or naïve about this. Let's look first at what has been written about policy-making and then move on to see this at work with some examples of the politics of health in the UK.

Democracy

The basis of political power in the UK and many other countries lies in the principle that the political party with the most elected candidates in parliament has a mandate to implement its policies. However governments regularly devise policies and actions that appear not to have widespread support from the public. The decision that UK forces would join the military invasion of Iraq in 2003 has been widely seen as the result of the strong belief of one individual, for example, and evoked mass demonstrations. While the origins of democracy in Greek society may have been delegative, that is as long as you were not a slave or a woman you could directly take part in decision-making, in today's far larger states we have representative democracy. By voting for a particular political candidate we invest our decision-making power in that individual for the period of their office. That arrangement may have become the norm but when it is mixed with more 'direct' forms of democracy such as membership votes and referenda, fault lines can appear. Currently two such examples are reverberating in the UK. The most extraordinary is the result of the UK referendum on membership of the

European Union undertaken on 23 June 2016. While most of the UK business sector, scientists, economic and banking advisers as well as the majority of MPs were supporting the 'remain' campaign and a coalition of far-right and careerist politicians steered the leave campaign with strong elements of racism, the result of the referendum was that the majority of voters expressed a wish for the country to leave the EU. One commentator described the shocked 'leavers' after the result as like 'the dog that got on the bus'. Many 'remainers', in disbelief, signed a petition for a re-run of the vote and claimed that those who voted leave were duped by false promises from the leave campaign. The decision opened up or rather revealed a shocking gulf between the establishment and large sections of the general public. At the heart of the remain consciousness was perhaps the unshakeable belief that they knew best.

The other problematic example of apparent democracy in action takes the form of the elections among the membership of the Labour party for that party's leader, also in 2016. Candidate Jeremy Corbyn, widely considered to sit at the party's left wing gained overwhelming support and claimed a significant mandate. However a great many Labour MPs refused to work with him for a mixture of political (they thought he was too left wing) and personal (they think him a poor leader) reasons, significantly undermining his position. Finally a fellow MP has been persuaded to stand against him in a new leadership contest but when the new leadership vote is run, it seems highly likely that Corbyn will be returned again on the basis of his popular support. As with the above example many Labour MPs and former prominent Labour figures seem to be saying to the party's (greatly expanded) membership that they know best when it comes to choosing a leader.

Democracy is a term with a self-evident value but its operation and its varieties show that the concept is complex and problematic.

Given the complexities of the democratic influence on politics let's go on to ask how is government policy made? There are a number of forces that influence politicians and policy-making.

Influencers

Success in politics involves knowing the difference between who you can afford to upset and who you can't. Politicians are surrounded by interest or pressure groups. They also have to respond to voters and, crucially, to attention in the media. Let's look at this source of influence first.

In the UK, as in most democratic countries, national newspapers express a spectrum of political views or orientations.[1] Politicians know that how issues are covered in newspapers can have a major effect on the popularity of their policies and their political careers. The most widely read newspaper in the UK, *The Sun*, has backed the winning party in general elections since 1979. The same newspaper also urged readers to vote for exit from the EU in the 2016 referendum. So politicians, despite protests to the contrary, may think twice before upsetting its owner billionaire Rupert Murdoch. The Leveson Inquiry into press ethics found close and problematic relationships between senior politicians and figures in the print media (Leveson The Right Honourable Lord Justice 2012). In evidence to the inquiry ex-prime minister Tony Blair described the sense of having to stay on favourable terms with a powerful press:

> [I]f you're a political leader and you have very powerful media groups and you fall out with one of those groups, the consequence is such that it really means that you then are effectively blocked from getting across your message.[2]

The popular press presents a constant backdrop to our lives, often full of threatening characters such as migrants trying to enter the UK (Gutteridege 2016) or cruel and uncaring nurses

---

1 This diversity can be overestimated as just three companies control nearly 70% of national newspaper circulation in the UK: Media Reform Coalition (2014).

2 See *Transcript of Morning Hearing*, 28 May 2012, p. 4 [pdf]. Available at: www.levesoninquiry.org.uk/wpcontent/uploads/2012/05/Transcript-of-Morning-Hearing-28-May-2012.pdf

reducing their patients to drinking water from flower vases (Matthews 2010).

Failures and scandals in the NHS make good news stories. So avoiding unwanted media coverage represents a driver of health policy for health ministers. They will want above all to be seen to be responding decisively to well-publicized crises such as the scandals of care at Stafford, even if informed commentators can see that their interventions may be un-thought through or counter-productive, or too late. The relationship between public opinion and the media is not straightforward but the two are related and politicians note that the communications they receive from constituents tend to reflect current headlines.

Pressure groups aim to influence political power, or, more specifically, the making of public policy (Kavanagh 2006). We can classify pressure groups in a number of ways. The first type of group is promotional, cause or attitude-based. We can include among them those campaigning for reform to abortion law, for example, and the 'think-tanks' representing views across the political spectrum. A second group would be sectional or interest groups. These would include the City of London representing the UK financial sector, occupational groups and trade unions. The most useful distinction, however, if we are trying to account for which groups have influence, is that between insider and outsider groups. Insider groups are those that have regular contact with policymakers in the relevant government department. They tend to have information and expertise the government needs and they speak with authority for their sector. And though their aims would be broadly aligned to government policy, they also have the power to veto policy, in theory at least. The medical royal colleges come to mind as this kind of insider. The Thatcher government (1979–1990) however, set on public sector reform, took a confrontational approach toward groups that represented public sector providers, as well as, of course, unions. For that government, these groups were part of the national problem of self-interest and resistance to change that it sought to defeat. Perhaps since then governments of both the 'right' and 'left' have expected resistance and disagreement from these groups toward their reforms. The most recent reorganization of the NHS, introduced by Andrew Lansley during 2011 and 2012 (see box above) seems to have encountered an unprecedented amount of opposition from the main medical and nursing organizations, resulting in them being excluded from key consultation meetings. Nevertheless those professions are represented by senior civil servants (the Chief Medical Officer and the Chief Nursing Officer) who have no alternative but to work cooperatively with ministers, trying to insert beneficial action for their professions into already existing government policy.

Science

It would be natural to think that governments look to the world of expertise to inform key decision-making. How do we best deal with HIV/AIDS or Ebola? What is the best treatment for Mad Cow Disease and how serious is the threat? How can we alleviate poverty? Is petrol better for the environment than diesel fuel? How does migration affect the UK economy? How would leaving the European Union affect nurse recruitment? Because science is a supposedly rational process, for some it would follow that science can have – or should have – an influence in a value-free way. The mechanisms of scientific influence are complex and those who study the topic agree that there is no simple link (Buse *et al.* 2005). Much depends on the networks and routes of influence that members of the scientific community have established with civil servants[3] who advise government ministers, a kind of 'policy community'. Key to influence is the perceived acceptability of the scientific advice. Even the scientific community's presentation of statistics on certain topics may be unwelcome. Classic examples of the length of time that scientific

---

3   The term 'civil servants' describes the array of administration and advice that government ministers use to support their work. Civil servants range from junior clerical or research staff to the figureheads such as the Chief Medical Officer. In theory they are apolitical posts as they have to work with whatever government is in office.

advice can take to affect policy are the evidence for the link between lung cancer and smoking and HIV/AIDS prevention. Epidemiological links had been found between smoking and lung cancer in the 1950s but policy action only began to be taken in the mid-1960s to alert the public to the risks and to control tobacco advertising on television. The first health warnings appeared on cigarette packets in 1971 (Berridge 2006). In the case of HIV/AIDS, Margaret Thatcher was said to be resistant to the suggestion of mass health education campaigns that explicitly mentioned anal intercourse. This was despite evidence of the time that anal sex had been linked with 85% of AIDS cases and guidance stemming from this evidence was considered an essential part of the health promotion message by the then chief medical officer (Milmo 2015). Rather later, but revealingly, during the campaign on UK European Union membership, MP and former education secretary Michael Gove in reply to warnings from economists about the dangers of leaving the EU remarked that the British public had 'had enough of experts' (Mance 2016). He made it explicit that politicians feel free to ignore scientific advice in pursuit of political objectives.

Ideology

Political parties and their members tend to have a set of beliefs and values regarding what society is, what would make a good society and the nature of the barriers to reaching this along with how these should be overcome. There are various definitions of the term ideology but let's call this organized set of beliefs by that name for the moment.

Sometimes these can be based on fundamental beliefs about human nature and motivation, for example about whether people are generally motivated by individual self-interest or by maintaining solidarity with others. Alongside this there can be some ambiguity between beliefs about how people are and how they could or should be. People *ought* to be encouraged or enabled to maximize their own interests, for example. These beliefs often underpin political policies, sometimes only implicitly.

Today we talk about the political 'right' and 'left'. This terminology originated during the French Revolution (1789–1799). The members of the country's National Assembly were divided into supporters of the king and supporters of the revolution. Supporters of the king began to sit to the right of the president, while supporters of the revolution sat to the left. Since then right wing has tended to refer to supporters of the establishment and left-wingers those who oppose and challenge it.

In more recent times (see section on neoliberalism) the left has been associated with collectivist approaches to the running of society while the right, often referred to as the New Right, has championed more individualized and perhaps individualistic values. It is sometimes linked with libertarian approaches. These range from the ethos behind the development of the Bitcoin currency in the desire to avoid reliance on large banking corporations, to the US movements that demand the right to carry firearms in public.

Ideology has been understood sometimes in ways that emphasize that it is something illusory, distorted or mystifying and sometimes as sets of ideas that organize social, cultural and economic life. The second use does not foreground the question of whether the ideas are true or not but rather emphasizes the impossibility that any cultural practice does not emerge from some set of presuppositions and values. Ideology does not have to be explicit or conscious to be effective. In fact it is most effective when it is not. I discuss Marx's idea of ideology in Chapter 8.

Neoliberalism and the market

Since the mid-1980s one particular ideology has dominated public policies in the UK, the United States and an increasing

range of countries. This is neoliberalism (Navarro 2007).
I summarized a neoliberal view of higher education in the
previous chapter but I will develop the main points here.
Neoliberalism, perhaps like all ideologies, presents itself as a
simple and unavoidable economic fact. Its origins are said to be
in Adam Smith's *The Wealth of Nations*, published in 1776
(Smith 1904). Smith argued that the wealth of a nation originates
not from the accumulation of wealth by the state at the expense
of its citizens or foreign powers, but as a result of the initiatives
and enterprise of private individuals (Clarke 2005). He believed
that free exchange between individuals was a transaction from
which both parties would benefit because no one would
voluntarily participate in a deal from which they would emerge
worse off. Restrictions on trade would only hinder this mutually
beneficial and wealth-creating activity.[4]

However, history, it is argued, soon revealed that the benefits
of free trade flowed overwhelmingly to the more economically
advanced and/or politically powerful party.

> While free trade brought prosperity to the most advanced
> producers, it imposed destitution on those who were unable
> to compete, provoking periodic crises in which less advanced
> producers were bankrupted, masses of people were thrown
> out of work and the trade of whole nations came to a
> standstill. This experience gave rise to demands for state
> protection for small producers and for the national indus-
> try of the productively less advanced countries. Small
> producers saw the source of their difficulties in the power
> of the bankers, who denied them access to the credit they
> needed to sustain themselves, while capitalists of less
> advanced countries sought tariff protection for their national
> industries. For the liberal political economists, of course,
> periodic crises and bankruptcy were part of the healthy

4   Low taxes have, in recent years, become part of a neoliberal framework
    because high tax rates are seen as a counter-incentive to entrepreneurialism
    and wealth generation and part of the state's interference in the economy.

operation of the market, the stick that accompanied the carrots offered to the more enterprising producers. The market was not just an economic, but also a moral force, penalising the idle and incompetent and rewarding the enterprising and hard-working, for the greater good of society as a whole.

(Clarke 2005 p. 2)

The neoliberal model was influential through much of the nineteenth century in Britain, supporting the growth of industrialization. Industrialization, however led to social ills of which child labour and the illnesses of poverty and overcrowding were prominent. A social reform movement grew in that century and continued in a fragmentary way until the end of World War Two, with the much-written-about formation of the UK National Health Service part of a comprehensive policy of welfarism. And it is to this as an example of a political intervention that we will now turn.

Policy examples: the creation of a welfare state in the UK

The use of policy by governments to achieve social ends is relatively recent. In the late nineteenth century many states had taken up responsibility for 'public goods' such as sanitation and public health but it was after World War Two, and then during the 1960s, especially in the United States, that they used social policy more actively to combat problems such as poverty or ill health. In 1948, shortly after the end of World War Two, the National Health Service was set up, by a Labour government elected in 1945, as part of a rise of humanism that swept Europe and North America in response to the horrors of the war.[5]

5   Social reformer William Beveridge (1879–1963), whose 1942 report on social insurance was one of the founding influences for the UK's welfare state, saw healthcare as crucial to the slaying of the five 'giants' ('want, disease, squalor, ignorance and idleness') in the post-World War Two reconstruction of Britain.

Its establishment was also an acknowledgement that the situation in which the poor relied on the services of charitable hospitals was no longer viable. The principle of the National Health Service was one of universal access and shared risk, being largely funded from taxation and free to those who used its services. After some debate, it was developed as a centralized (rather than locally organized) scheme. However, any insurance-based system of healthcare needs to solve several major problems (Strong and Robinson 1990). Probably the most pressing is the open-ended nature of healthcare. This has consequences for the financial sustainability of the system as a whole, partly because medical-technological and pharmaceutical development mean healthcare costs are likely to be continually rising, potentially at an exponential rate. If it was ever assumed in the early days of the NHS that the service would abolish ill health and then could be closed down, the opposite has occurred. Coupled with a growing range of increasingly expensive treatment options, more of the population is living longer and older people tend to be greater users of the service. The population as a whole is said to have higher expectations of healthcare. Add to this the tendency of powerful professional monopolies to expand their services and encourage their use, alongside pharmaceutical companies looking for sales, then we have a set of inbuilt problems that politicians of different political backgrounds have grappled with ever since.

Healthcare as a market

In January 1989 the Margaret Thatcher government announced a radical reform of the NHS. With advice from a leading North American health economist,[6] and with experienced politician Kenneth Clarke as health secretary, the white paper Working for Patients (Department of Health 1989) set out the government's solution to increasing costs within the service.

6   Alain Enthoven.

White papers are policy documents produced by the government that present their proposals for future legislation. White Papers are often published as so-called 'Command Papers' and may include a draft version of a Bill that is being planned. This provides a basis for further consultation and discussion with interested or affected groups and allows final changes to be made before a Bill is formally presented to parliament.

(www.parliament.uk/site-information/
glossary/white-paper/)

Although there were other aspects to the changes, in this summary I will concentrate on how the white paper proposed to incentivize those within the system to deliver more patient-centred, efficiently produced healthcare. The solution was to turn the collectivist state provision of healthcare into a market. How could this possibly be done when individuals had to rely almost entirely on the knowledge of clinicians to tell them what they needed, when in most areas there would be only limited choice in terms of treatment, especially in emergencies and when General Practitioners rather than patients themselves made choices in terms of tests and treatments?

The first step was to 'split' the NHS into 'purchasers' and 'providers'. Purchasers – the existing health authorities – received funds to pay for healthcare for their local populations. The second was to enable volunteering NHS providers, whether hospitals, community services or combinations of the two to apply for self-governing status – so-called NHS trusts with freedoms to borrow money and to set their own staff terms and conditions – though there were certain core services that they had to provide. The third was to allow General Practices with 11,000 or more patients (subsequently reduced) to apply to be given their own budgets to cover staff costs, medicines prescribing and a particular range of hospital services. The idea was that money would follow the patient through the system. From a neoliberal point of view, NHS providers would be incentivized to produce services that patients were satisfied with and which were cheaper than 'competitors'. GPs and health authorities would purchase more of these services while less flexible and less efficient providers would either catch up or, in theory, go out of business – perhaps be taken over by the successful trusts. Restrictions on commissioning services from the private sector were also loosened. There were unanswered questions, however, about the public desirability of such instability in local healthcare provision and whether certain groups of high-cost patients would be disadvantaged because providers might be reluctant to provide these complex and costly services.

The medical profession fiercely opposed the changes and the speed of introduction. In reality the 'market' needed to have many built-in protections, regulations, audits and restrictions so that many referred to this as a 'quasi-market' or, less kindly, as a 'pseudo-market'. The result was mixed and both 'sides' of the argument found evidence to support their position. Some claimed that the spirit of altruism that once characterized the service was lost in the face of a 'business ethos', while some studies seemed to show that fund-holding GPs had obtained better services for their patients (Brindle 1995, Audit Commission 1996). As with most political changes, particularly the many reorganizations of the NHS, the complexity of the context and the many possible ways of measuring 'improvement' mean it is hard to give one verdict on the internal market. We can see it however as a bold experiment in applying neoliberal principles to a complex and highly visible public service.

Professions are the problem: nursing as a policy instrument

An incoming Labour administration abolished the internal market in 1997, saving, it said, '£1 billion on red tape and putting that money into frontline patient care' (Department of Health 1997). Although it set about addressing the inequalities of care that had resulted from the variation in GP fundholding across the country, certain features of Conservative policy were here to stay. These were private sector involvement, a concern for the assessment of quality, peer review, central government direction, performance reporting, accountability, competition, trusts, patient choice and payment by results (Dixon 2008). The years of Labour's rule saw five secretaries of state for health, from 1998 to 2007, each with their different personal approach and political standpoint. However, one strong theme that emerged from the beginning of the Blair years is that of 'modernization' and white papers reflected this emphasis. And New Labour, more than any other administration, used nursing to achieve this policy objective. The idea was that 'modernization' could be achieved by reducing professional demarcation (barriers between what one professional group was allowed to do and another) that was seen as old-fashioned and rigid as well as poor for patient experience. New Labour strategy enabled the nursing profession to move onto territory previously occupied by medicine. These features can be seen in the following summary of policy that affected nursing.

The Nurse-led NHS Direct: announced in *The New NHS Modern Dependable* (Department of Health 1997). This telephone service was intended to reduce GP and hospital emergency department work and was described as creating a new career opportunity for nurses. It was closed down in 2014.

Nurse Consultant posts: these were first proposed in *Making a Difference* published in 1999 (Department of Health 1999). The document set out to deliver two messages, that nurses were a valued part of the workforce and that they should be more influential on care. Nurse consultants could provide a stronger focus for clinical leadership along with 'modernized' roles for nurses.

Modern Matrons: *The NHS Plan* (Department of Health 2000) promoted a new clinical nursing leader, the 'Modern Matron', who would be given authority to deal with ward level problems that had dominated in the media such as lack of cleanliness and hospital acquired infection.

'Ten key roles' for nurses were announced by the Chief Nursing Officer in England (Department of Health 2000). Many

of these key roles were previously undertaken by doctors. This included expansions to nurse prescribing.

On the face of it, and in a way are these, exciting new ventures for nurses. However we can see these initiatives as driven, not by the profession itself because according to word at the time some of the initiatives came as a surprise to the profession, but by the need to meet changing NHS political pressures and priorities. For example in 2000 and 2001 when patient waiting lists were causing controversy *The NHS Plan CNO's message to nurses* (March 2001) focussed on how new nursing roles could progress patients' journeys through the healthcare system. Nurses would reduce waiting and improve access to the system by providing additional points of access. Nursing role substitution for doctors was also promoted as a mechanism for addressing another key government objective to do with increasing patient choice. The CNO and Department of Health presented new nursing roles in walk-in centres and GP surgeries, along with nurse-led clinics in specialities such as gastroscopy, as nursing's specific contribution to this major objective.

Post-Francis, post-everything

I cannot end a chapter on politics and politicians without, even briefly, bringing us up to the present day, the time of writing. Not for the first time, as we have seen, the NHS is financially in trouble. Austerity budgets from the Conservative (ex-) chancellor George Osborne have featured some drastic cuts to NHS spending including an estimated 20% cut to the public health budget (Stone 2015), reductions of £1.1billion to NHS repairs (Broomfield 2016) and '£650 million in secret cuts' to the NHS (Stone 2016). Many NHS trusts are in deficit and there were an estimated 20,000 unfilled nursing posts in 2013 (Ford 2013). There are limits on agency spending for NHS employers and, in the light of the problems raised by the Francis and other reports critical of nursing (Cavendish 2013, Francis 2013b, Keogh 2013), NICE issued guidelines in 2014 on safe staffing for nursing in some settings, and then announced it was no longer working on the project (Lintern 2015).

What nurses can do

Many nurses and students feel like Kevin whose uncertainty about whether to leave the profession or to try to get a position of influence opened this chapter. I have tried to show how the forces that drive politics and politicians have had a major and continuing impact on the daily work of nurses. It was a political idea to develop the NHS and politicians since have used it to act out their ideologies and to make a stamp on this popular and highly visible part of the public sector. The driver for their attention has been a combination of the service's apparently insatiable appetite for cash and its high media visibility, both at local and national level. Politicians of all major parties are keen to state their commitment to its principles but many commentators foresee its imminent demise through creeping privatization. Nurses, as well as doctors and other clinical professionals can feel like footballs being kicked around by opposing teams. Nurses have expressed a sense of injustice at the hands of politicians generally, claiming that they are expected to deliver caring services while politicians do not 'care' for them and their working conditions. There is even a poem about this that resonated with the RCN Congress when it was recited in 2013.[7]

So what does this mean in relation to critical resilience, the topic of this book? I think having an understanding of the mechanisms of politics – at least those that can be known – may do two things. It might highlight our awareness of the problems and contradictions in policy and, from certain perspectives, highlight our sense of elements of injustice enacted in policy. But it is also important to join with others to focus our energies on understanding and analysing events and their causes rather than surrendering to a feeling of generalized martyrdom. I think Kevin is right: our choice is between contributing to making the work of nursing better or to 'vote with our feet', leave and do something different.

---

7   The poet is Molly Case who was at the time a student nurse. The recitation and, perhaps more importantly, the response from around four thousand nurses is at www.youtube.com/watch?v=XOCda6OiYpg.

If you are a student nurse you have a foot in two different cultures: the university and the National Health Service. Although much is made of their differences they have a lot in common. They are both part of the public sector – funded by and ultimately controlled by the government which is, in turn, funded and ultimately controlled by the public. Because of this their working budgets are determined in a way that is largely outside of their control and hence they are vulnerable to the ideologies of and contingencies facing the government of the day. They both face considerable external scrutiny and control of their performance and organization. And although senior figures in each sector are financially well rewarded, it is often said that those who decide to work in universities and the health service do so because they are motivated to make a positive difference to the lives of those they deal with, an orientation to values beyond the walls of their particular employing organization. These values might be the values of a profession or of a historical intellectual movement. Much of the tension you might experience in the workplace is likely to be a result of that dual identity: member of a profession as well as salaried employee of a particular organization. If you are in the middle of a nursing degree you have a third identity – that of a university student, and from 2017, one that shells out £9,000 a year for the privilege.

To be a critically resilient student nurse you need to know something about what makes NHS organizations tick as well as the inside story of the university. To understand something of this can help explain the events and behaviour you encounter from day to day at work and in study. In the previous chapter I talked about health policy at the level of governments. In this chapter I am looking at organizations. Those employed in universities or in senior NHS roles will be all too familiar with much of the content of this chapter. Those who are students or, perhaps, relatively junior workers may find it an eye-opener.

Pros and cons of being in the university

In Chapter 5 I discussed how students of nursing and those that teach them found their way into universities. Although some in nursing are not convinced this was the right move, the benefits of university-based education outweigh the problems. The benefits, I suggest, are: having a recognized level of qualification that can be accepted by employers in other sectors; sharing an environment with students taking different courses and the accompanying opportunity for gaining a wider understanding of different perspectives; having easier access to specialist lecturers; and the development of courses that reflect the kind of skills that nurses need in order to work in the complex NHS environment. But there are disadvantages that impact on students and these stem from the separation of lecturers from the clinical setting. Because lecturers are employed by and based in universities they rely on other people to support students in the clinic and there is potential for a kind of drifting apart in priorities and sensibilities between lecturers and nurses still in clinical practice. Different settings have developed different solutions to this separation in the form of individuals whose job it is to keep good connections between the university and the clinic such as practice education teachers and link lecturers. But there are perhaps not enough people employed in these roles and one 'link' lecturer can have a large number of different clinical areas to keep links with. The other weakness is that if lecturers are educated and paid to lecture, devise curricula and assess academic work, the same is expected from those in the clinical setting who teach and assess clinical skills – and these are the mentors. Mentors, as any student reading this will know, play a vital part in nurse education. They teach and assess, sometimes making the decision whether individual students are of the right standard to be added to the nursing register and act as role models for students. They do this with little specific preparation or reward and they do it alongside a normal clinical workload, 'with other patients to look after' as one student in one of my focus groups

1   This student and others felt as dependent as the sick patients they witnessed and identified with them. This identification is perhaps one reason why students are highly sensitized to deficiencies in patient care, particularly around attitude and a failure to take the time to listen to patients expressing their needs.

put it in a Freudian slip.[1] That this is done with any kind of success is a testament to mentors and students for being flexible. However, it is not an ideal design – in fact you could call it education on the cheap – and probably the major topic raised in focus groups I have run with students over the years has been dissatisfaction and frustration with mentors. Some students blame individual mentors and are very vocal about their treatment and their mentor's moral deficiencies. Others tell stories of changing their opinion when, after some workload alteration, their mentors have a miraculous personality change and become friendly and helpful. This is a prime example of what a difference an awareness of the structural causes of day-to-day problems can make.

So, the situation, particularly in the clinical setting, is problematic by design and inadequately addressed by policymakers. This puts individuals under sustained pressure as staff 'cope' with demands that are close to impossible to meet so, along with clinical skills, student nurses learn something rather negative about nursing culture. One outcome of any situation where there is sustained pressure can be seen in eruptions of violence and bullying. I will end this chapter with one of the most important parts of this book, a critical approach to dealing with bullying in the workplace. But first, by way of an essential introduction, more on the forces that influence day-to-day experience.

Structural forces on university nursing

If you really want to understand how an organization works and make sense of the actions its members take that affect you, you need to know what incentives and penalties it faces. And in recent years governments have set up an increasing number of – basically financial – controls for universities, as well as the NHS which we will discuss next, to encourage the particular kind of activity it wants to see. In higher education these take the form of regular formal assessments of particular types of activity, measured at the level of the university as a whole, assigned a numerical score and usually given the name 'quality': 'teaching quality' or 'research quality' to name the most significant. Universities invest considerable hours and efforts preparing for these exercises because the outcomes can make available huge amounts of cash if they do well. A good result can also add to a university's reputation. Reputation though is prized because it in turn brings more students, and they bring more funding. As I write, the government are proposing a new exercise, the Teaching Excellence Framework, in order to measure the quality of university teaching and reward those universities that do well by granting them permission to raise their tuition fees higher than the current £9,000 per year.[2] Then there is the annual National Student Survey (NSS), a survey commissioned by the Higher Education Funding Councils in the UK, where students are asked 23 questions relating to their experiences at their university. The results allow the funding councils to publish a league table of universities. Moving up or down even a few places becomes an event of major scrutiny for university managers and their staff. Finally there are incentives and penalties attached to the regular processes that the university engages in such as recruitment, operating for example by governments placing a limit on the number of recruited students allowed in the sector, or by removing that cap, or by funding every type of course or removing funding for particular areas. If you are not a member of staff at such an institution it is probably hard to be aware of the way that such exercises create pressure that usually starts, as in most organizations, with the most senior figures and is passed down through levels of management with varying degrees of genuine incentive to improve on the one hand and working out ways of getting a good score on the other. Please don't misunderstand the point I am making about this. My point is not that these mechanisms distract university employees like the lecturers you deal with from their real work, but that incentives have a strange way of becoming detached from the things that they are meant to be

2   See http://monitor.icef.com/2015/11/british-government-proposes-major-higher-education-reform-package/ for a brief summary of the proposals contained in the green paper.

about. If student experience is being measured by some external body who can penalize you for getting it wrong, then paradoxically your attention and anxiety become focussed on avoiding the penalty and not any more on student experience, anti-intuitive as this sounds.[3]

Added to this, nursing education, like other professional courses (teaching and social work for example) is closely monitored by a number of external organizations. One is the body that currently commissions universities to train nursing students (as well as other non-medical professionals), Health Education England (HEE). HEE was set up in 2012 and has 13 regional offices, three of these for different parts of London. It makes final decisions about the numbers of students that it commissions, taking into account individual NHS trusts' annual workforce plans and the overall budget from the Department of Health, which has effectively put a limit on the maximum number recruited. In reality the number of student places that are commissioned rises and falls depending on the current financial state of the NHS. Each individual university has been set targets for recruitment for the different branches of nursing and those responsible for recruitment have to make a number of offers to prospective students knowing that not all will be accepted. It is like throwing a paper dart into a crosswind. There are financial implications for over or under recruiting so it is important to get it right. From 2017, however, as I have previously mentioned, the government plan to change this approach. Instead of giving a budget for tuition and clinical placement costs for students, prospective nurse students will have to take loans from the Student Loan Company and the only limit on the number of students in training will be universities' capacity – physical space to teach and numbers of staff to do it – and the availability of clinical placements. HEE say they will continue to manage clinical placements and implement a workforce plan for the NHS.

3   Think of how the 4-hour waiting time limit in hospital emergency departments affects decision-making in that setting. See later section on the impact of this target.

If you are a new student nurse who started a course in 2017, don't be surprised to see some puzzled faces as university personnel and NHS staff try to work out how this change can be made to work. I have mentioned elsewhere that the proposal has met with strong resistance from student organizations and mixed responses from the nursing profession.

The other body that shapes the way that universities teach student nurses is the NMC, the profession's regulator. Professional regulators today make it very clear that their overriding priority is to protect the public. NMC publicity repeats this so many times that it is impossible to miss. Previous versions of today's NMC have been successively criticized by government-commissioned inquiries for being too friendly to the profession. Today's NMC is strongly influenced by the state who have, over the years, rebalanced the regulator's governing body in favour of lay members (e.g. JM Consulting Ltd. 1998, Ford 2012). Its current Chief Executive has a legal rather than a nursing background. A key principle of a profession is that the route of entry into it is strictly controlled by the profession itself. The NMC keeps a register of qualified nurses but also devises standards for nurse and midwifery education that, it says, shape the content and design of nursing and midwifery programmes (see www.nmc.org.uk/education/our-role-in-education/). Every course leading to registration has to be approved by the NMC

Regulators such as the NMC have to balance the interests of three different groups: their own members whose professional fees pay their bills, the public who look to these bodies to protect them against poor practice and the government who hold, in theory at least, final power over them. This assumption that the regulatory bodies make decisions in the interests of the public, rather than their membership, differentiates them from professional associations like the Royal College of Nursing (RCN) or British Medical Association (BMA).

and institutions that run them have also to be approved. The NMC visits institutions and carries out monitoring reviews that include gathering the views of students and service users. Although the NMC describes its approach as intended to enable innovation in nurse education, many nurse educators see the influence of the NMC as overall a conservative one in terms of their own desires to devise progressive courses.

How the NHS workplace works

Students spend half of their course in clinical settings and this is mainly, though not entirely, in NHS trusts. Political forces and budget constraints have a huge impact on these organizations and they need very committed and talented management to stay focussed on delivering good quality care to patients and clients while enabling a supportive and vibrant workplace for employees.

If you are a student you will know only too well that your experience both personally and in terms of learning varies between different organizations and between different parts of the same organization. The culture of any given unit depends on a combination of factors: top level leadership, the support or otherwise of middle management, overall budgets, relationships with medical staff and other professional groups, ward-based leadership, team dynamics and patient characteristics. When all of these go well then professional work can flourish but problems with any component higher up can cause anxiety that spreads down through the organizational hierarchy. And students, albeit unofficially, are at the bottom end of this order.

It is important to understand the less tangible but nevertheless highly pervasive forces that determine organizational culture. I introduced neoliberalism in other places in this book but want to move on this chapter by talking about neoliberalism's mode of operation in the public sector, managerialism. Traditional ideas of profession do not sit well with neoliberalism's belief in the free market. A profession seems too much like a group with a monopoly of an area of work that can stifle competition and innovation, both of which are seen as typical free market forces that create wealth. The Thatcher government looked to techniques from commerce to address the lack of accountability and responsiveness that it saw as typical of medicine (there were few similar concerns about nursing) (Strong and Robinson 1990). It introduced general management. This was the alternative to a previous situation where any given NHS hospital for example would have three separate lines of hierarchy: medical, nursing and administrative, with the tacit assumption that it was doctors who were in charge. The idea was that a good general manager did not need specific medical or nursing know-how to manage a hospital well. More important was the ability to set objectives, make them happen and ensure accountability. In fact a general manager was less likely to push for ever-expanding services in the way that senior medical figures might. The plan led to a great deal of opposition from the nursing and medical organizations along the predictable line of argument that managers without specialist professional backgrounds could not possibly know how a service should be run or what was best for patients. At the risk of oversimplifying, the single challenge for governments – and not just for Margaret Thatcher's administration – was how to get doctors to do what they wanted.

Some commentators said that little changed after general management but the direction was set and successive reforms and restructures including the 'internal market' (see Chapter 6) and mechanisms of measurement introduced by the Tony Blair government have definitely shifted the atmosphere if not the ethos of the NHS. Activity is measured, norms are set and those units or even individuals who perform poorly on these measures can be identified and penalized. As mentioned before, targets and incentives can give rise to 'unintended' but quite predicable consequences. An investigation by the group Dr Foster identified the way that some NHS trusts instigated practices aimed at avoiding penalties for missing targets that negatively affected patient care.

> These include patients being kept in ambulances outside hospital to delay the 'clock starting' on the waiting time, and evidence that patients are most likely to be admitted

just before they have been waiting four hours, suggesting that some doctors may be admitting unnecessarily, in order to avoid target breaches.

(Cooper 2015)

The same report went on to claim that pressure to hit targets was also a contributor to workplace bullying in the NHS citing an example of a trust that was under investigation following allegations of manipulated waiting list data. The reduction of waiting times had been a key element of New Labour's health policy so it was keen to be seen to be successful in this very visible area of health policy. Improvements in this, and other 'targeted' areas occurred alongside gaming, resource allocation away from other areas, falsification and bullying.

What motivates you in your work? Why did you decide to become a nurse or a lecturer? Neoliberal governments are attempting to replace the range of different motivations in varying areas of work with a single type of motivation that is financial. So, perhaps to oversimplify, while NHS staff are motivated by a desire to help people in sickness, and those in universities are motivated by intellectual development and broadening the minds of university students, governments apply the single motivating principle of financial incentives and penalties to individuals who identify with entirely different principles. Organizations appoint managers who may not share these professional values but do understand the penalties and incentives. No wonder there is a sense of jarring in both sectors, a sense of jarring which a student would experience without, perhaps, knowing its political origin.

What to do about bullying at work or at college

Feeling that you are being bullied at work or at college is, excuse my language, shit. It can turn you from a confident and good-humoured professional practitioner or motivated student into a self-doubting mess, unable to sleep or make decisions. Outsiders to nursing and healthcare always notice how hierarchical both are. The people who don't need reminding about hierarchies are generally those near the bottom. Hierarchies are great places for bullies. There is no more urgent time for critical resilience than when you are being bullied. In this section I want to talk first about structural pressures that can play on individuals' weaknesses and bring out bullying behaviour and then what you can do if you feel you are being bullied. Structural explanations do not excuse a bully's behaviour but they can help us to feel slightly more informed and in control in a difficult and charged situation.

When organizations – NHS trusts or universities – have to operate with reducing budgets or to continue to operate with increasing costs with budgets that do not keep up, or have to operate with threats of budget cuts, there is bound to be an impact. The most humane and conscientious managers may end up making unpalatable decisions in the almost impossible position of having to maintain an acceptable level of service with inadequate budgets. Detecting inefficiency and waste can only go so far and in any case is often a matter of judgement – is a 15-minute patient appointment a waste of 10 of those minutes, for example? Senior managers restructure their organizations to try to wipe off costs. In reorganizations it is often middle level managers, in universities deans and heads of schools and their deputies who are made redundant or moved to other less preferable posts. In NHS trusts wards or units can be merged to save the salary of a ward manager or two. In the account books this can solve problems, usually only temporally, but in people's lives there is nearly always an effect. Both suddenly losing your income and position as well as anxiety about this being about to happen can alter people's behaviour, sometimes dramatically. It would be surprising if it did not. Optimistically adversity might draw people together and increase solidarity but often the opposite happens. Cultures of uncertainty, anxiety, fear and resentment can develop. The well-known events at Stafford Hospital show graphically how a senior management under financial pressure gradually corrupted morale and professional practice throughout the whole organization producing intimidated middle managers and despairing and cynical nursing and medical staff. A report from researchers at Cranfield School of Management that commented on the situation at Stafford pays particular attention to the predicament of middle managers in 'low-trust – low-autonomy' environments (Buchanan *et al.* 2013).[4] When middle managers are placed under pressure or feel they have no control over decision-making that involves their own staff and services such pressures can seep into the most vulnerable places in their psyche. Those with a vulnerability to a sense of powerlessness can become resentful and embittered. Those who have a reduced repertoire of responses can turn to macho and dictatorial approaches as a way of coping with their own insecurities about their status and position. Now imagine you arrive one morning at their office with a query that is important to your work.

In a review of bullying at work, the British Psychological Society tells us that the majority of bullying is done by managers and that younger workers who may be unaware of their workplace rights, as well as members of ethnic minorities, are the most vulnerable to bullying (Cartwright and Cooper 2007). Research has consistently shown that the incidence of bullying is higher in the public than the private sector and this is often attributed to the relentless amount of change and increased performance pressures that public sector employees have experienced in recent years (Hoel and Cooper 2000). Psychologists

4   See a short, readable summary of the conclusions of this research at the Cranfield website www.som.cranfield.ac.uk/som/p19554/Think-Cranfield/Think-Cranfield-2013/April-2013/Mid-Staffordshire-hospital-making-the-right-changes

have identified some of the apparent individual characteristics of bullies, e.g. unresolved conflicts, poor social skills as well as personal biases and prejudices; however, they increasingly emphasize the link between bullying and work setting with stressful and changing environments, along with high workload being particularly associated with bullying. Anxieties about their own status and future can cause some individuals to become self-absorbed with their own standing and to be excessively critical of the work of others (Cartwright and Cooper 2007). My own research into the management of (so-called) poor performance in nursing showed that some of what might be considered overreaction to apparent performance issues was carried out by inexperienced managers keen to be seen to be reacting adequately (Traynor *et al.* 2013).

Action you can take

The TUC (Trades Union Congress) when speaking about bullying at work reminds us that:

> Employers have a duty under the Health and Safety at Work Act 1974 to ensure the health, safety and welfare of their employees. If they do not do this they are breaching an individual's contract of employment. It may also be a breach of sexual harassment and racial discrimination legislation, and the bully could well be guilty of harassment. Employers and/or the bully may find themselves facing fines, compensation and in some cases even a jail sentence.
>
> (www.tuc.org.uk/workplace-issues/health-
> and-safety/bullying/bullied-work-dont-
> suffer-silence)

The NHS, as well as the major health trade unions, offer guidance to anyone who feels they are being bullied at work. They have the same general contents which I will summarize and comment on:

Do not suffer alone. Speak to a friendly colleague and/or your trade union representative, or if you are a student, to a link lecturer or tutor. While I have heard the view that complaints to tutors are ineffective, the key principle is not to let yourself be isolated and intimidated or so ashamed that you dare not tell others what is happening. Our imaginations can get out of control and make a difficult situation feel overwhelming. Talking to others is highly likely to give us a welcome reality check.

Speak to the bully. This advice is given on the grounds that sometimes bullying is unintentional and that feedback can genuinely open the eyes of the person bullying you. The key would be to stay calm, polite and give examples of the behaviour that you do not like. It is possible that some bullies retreat from people who do not take on a victim role. This may prove effective. If there has been some element of genuine misunderstanding or miscommunication this could clear the air, for example it is possible that someone's clumsy attempt at relationship-forming humour may be received as belittling or insulting. However, there are plenty of situations, for example in NHS and university hierarchies where bullying is done by your manager or supervisor where this is just not feasible. Some advise that if you are being bullied by your manager you should speak to that manager's manager. However, this could be a high-risk strategy. It is not far-fetched to think that managers may tend to support each other under perceived attack from troublesome subordinates. If you do not feel safe with this course of action perhaps another individual placed in another part of the relevant organization may be more appropriate to listen and take suitable action. Do not agree to meetings called by the person bullying you without first asking exactly what the meeting is about and its status e.g. whether it is a disciplinary meeting. Take a representative or colleague with you, take notes in the meeting and do not agree to any suggestion made by the bully without first taking advice. As all the advice says, stay calm and, if you can, emotionally unengaged.

Keep a diary or other record of the events that you identify as bullying. Record, if you can, actual words spoken and the tone e.g. a raised voice, sarcasm or irritation along with times and dates. Make a note of emails you may have sent that were not replied to or phone messages that you have left that were not returned. This could prove useful evidence if you decide to take the matter further. Not replying to your messages can be part of the bully's technique.

Get advice from a trade union representative or legal adviser. Perhaps you have access through friendships or family contact with someone willing to give initially informal advice. It can be effective to then communicate, preferably in some written way, with those in the organization who you feel are bullying you stating explicitly what they (the bullies) have said, pointing out any inconsistencies with organizational policies, for example disciplinary or performance policies and asking for clarification. It is not unusual for managers or those in authority over you to hint at actions in face to face meetings that have no place in the organization's formal procedures. To point this out and ask for clarification is highly likely to silence bullies who rely on being able to intimidate victims.

The key to resilience in this situation is to *understand the character of what is happening* i.e. this is workplace bullying and that it is widespread, unacceptable and, depending on the nature of the bullying, possibly illegal. You do not have to justify yourself morally. It does not cast your character into doubt. It does not cast your competence into doubt. You do not have to consider leaving your course or resigning from your job, though this is often people's first reaction. It is far better for self-esteem to challenge and stand up. It can be surprising how one act of resistance from you can have a huge effect.

If all of these actions fail to change your situation then it could be time to move to new ground where you will be appreciated and flourish. You could at the same time consider counselling, therapy or analysis or making contact with groups of people in similar situations, not as act of weakness but as acknowledgement of trauma and as a promise to yourself to grow from adversity. Remember, this is a book about resilience.

Being a student and being a worker is not all bad! But it does happen in a context, a context that goes all the way from your colleagues and manager to the secretary of state for health or for education. In the next chapter I will set out a simple framework of the theories that go under the name of critical.

Chapter 8

Critical resilience and critical theory

This book is based on theory: this is no cause for alarm; this chapter provides an introduction to the difference between theory and common sense and how looking through theoretical glasses can make the world appear very different. I argue that theory can be liberating and empowering. This chapter looks at theoretical work that has gone under the name of critical including critical theory and I also talk about critical practice. Finally I offer some suggestions to where and how you can find out more.

In the 1988 film *They Live*, directed by John Carpenter, the hero, John Nada, a young drifter travelling the United States looking for work discovers in an abandoned church a dusty box of old sunglasses. But when he puts these apparently ordinary glasses on he has a shocking surprise. Through them the large and colourful advertising hoardings for washing powder or for holidays in the sun become sinister black and white subliminal messages such as 'Obey', 'Conform', 'Sleep'. He also sees that certain apparently normal humans are in reality aliens with skull-like faces who have penetrated society and hold some of its most powerful positions. Nada discovers a small group of other humans who also have access to the sunglasses

and the knowledge they bring. He joins with them in a
battle against these aliens.[1]

'Critical' is the first word of this book's title. When I place it in
front of 'resilience' everything is put into question. The whole
idea of the solution becomes a problem. This is not just
mischievousness on my part but an attempt to work within a
tradition and that tradition sometimes goes by the name of
'critical' or critical theory. The latter – critical theory – has a
specific origin and I want to spend some time in this chapter
talking about this. If there is one message from this chapter it
is this: theory can lead to a new self-awareness that can
contribute to a force for change.

What was there before theory?

Most theory is a reaction against something and sometimes that
'something' is explicit. Post-modernism is a reaction to
'modernism' or 'modernity'; post-structuralism a reaction to
structuralism. Critical theory was described and promoted as a
reaction to 'traditional' theory. Before I go further it is important
to understand two things. First, what I described as 'a reaction
to' often involves the paradox of a rejection of a previous theory
but at the same time an intensification of its insights or method,
a pushing further of its implications. Second, sometimes the
theory that is being overthrown did not necessarily exist as a
coherent named theory or movement. Criticisms of 'positivism'
are familiar in nursing texts about research but there were no

1 This movie is discussed by Slavoj Žižek in the film 'The Pervert's Guide to
   Ideology'. Currently you can see an excerpt from the Guide about *They
   Live* at www.youtube.com/watch?v=18qD9hmU9xg. The sunglasses are
   clearly a mechanism that allows the wearer to 'see through' ideology – a
   little like this book. Roll it into a tube and look through it but be prepared
   for what you see.

university Departments of Positivism (as far as I know) nor banner-waving positivists or at least there were none until the critiques came along.[2]

The Frankfurt School

The notion of critical theory was developed and defined by German sociologist Max Horkheimer (1895–1973), one of the founders of the Frankfurt School or the Institute for Social Research established in 1923 in Germany. In his 1937 essay *Traditional and Critical Theory* Horkheimer identified critical theory as a social theory orientated toward critiquing and changing society. Echoing Karl Marx's claim about philosophy, he contrasted critical theory with traditional theoretical work that satisfied itself with merely understanding or explaining society. However, Horkheimer differentiated the work of the Frankfurt School from classic Marxist theory identifying what he saw as the latter's covert positivism and authoritarianism in its strong claim to be scientific.

For Horkheimer (1972) traditional research takes place in a social and economic context that makes that work possible but can itself be overlooked by researchers despite their claim to involvement in a kind of project whose only framework is good science. This makes them complicit in society's interests:

> The scholar and his science are incorporated into the apparatus of society; his achievements are a factor in the conservation and continuous renewal of the existing state of affairs, no matter what fine names he gives to what he does.
> (p. 196)[3]

2 Yes, I know there were the Logical Positivists known as the Vienna Circle working in the late 1920s but I am not certain that they ever referred to themselves as 'positivists'.
3 Many since have developed this line of thought including those involved in Science and Technology Studies (STS). See for example one seminal work that shows laboratory scientists involved in highly entrepreneurial activity: Latour (1987).

Critical theory, at least in Horkheimer's formulation, rejects the positivist claim that knowledge built up through the collection of verifiable empirical facts becomes a *mirror* of reality. He goes on to make the argument for a critical scepticism:

> The world which is given to the individual and which he must accept and take into account is, in its present and continuing form, a product of the activity of society as a whole. The objects we perceive in our surroundings – cities, villages, fields, and woods – bear the mark of having been worked on by man. It is not only in clothing and appearance, in outward form and emotional make-up that men are the product of history. Even the way they see and hear is inseparable from the social life-process as it has evolved over the millennia. The facts which our senses present to us are socially preformed in two ways: through the histor-ical character of the object perceived and through the historical character of the perceiving organ. Both are not simply natural.
>
> (p. 200)

Critical theory therefore abandons a naïve conception of knowledge as impartial. Since researchers themselves are not disembodied entities, knowledge can only be obtained from within a society of interdependent individuals. The critical scholar must not become complicit in society's oppression:

> Although [critical research] emerges from the social structure, its purpose is not, either in its conscious intention or in its objective significance, the better functioning of any element in the structure. On the contrary, it is suspicious of the very categories of better, useful, appropriate, productive, and valuable, as these are understood in the present order, and refuses to take them as non-scientific presuppositions about which one can do nothing.
>
> (p. 207)

A critical researcher would ask in whose interests are projects that, in the case of this book, supposedly increase the resilience of subjects, whether 'disadvantaged' youth or hard-pressed nurses. Horkheimer goes so far as to suggest that there is likely to be some hostility to critical theory because it represents a threat to those who have come to accept their relatively subordinate position in bourgeois society:

> The demand therefore for a positive outlook and for acceptance of a subordinate position threatens, even in progressive sectors of society, to overwhelm any openness to theory.
>
> (p. 233)

The critical theorists researched a wide range of social, political, philosophical, psychoanalytic and cultural topics and built up an extensive body of work ranging from empirical studies to philosophical theorization. The richness and diversity of the Institute's work is its strength. In addition to Max Horkheimer a number of other influential writers have been associated with the Frankfurt School: Georg Lukacs (1885–1971), known for his writings on power; psychoanalyst Erich Fromm (1900–1980); psychologist Kurt Lewin (1890–1947), who developed action research and studied group communication; Herbert Marcuse (1898–1979), who developed a vision of the power of critical thought and studies of student counter-culture in the 1960s; Walter Benjamin (1892–1940), who studied literature and mass culture and Jürgen Habermas, known for his work on communication and consensus in society (see Habermas 1984).

In 1933, with the rise of the Nazis in Germany, the Institute was forced to close and its various members made their way to the United States[4] where they formed a new institute affiliated to Columbia University in New York. They continued, for a time, to publish in German, returning to what had become West Germany after the end of World War Two.

---

4 Only Walter Benjamin refused to leave Europe and, while attempting to cross the border between France and Spain in 1940, committed suicide.

Marxism

As you have seen, the critical theorists took as their departure Marxist theory. So for readers who are unfamiliar with it, I will set out the bare bones of Marx's economic theory.[5]

Marx (1818–1883) developed his theory in collaboration with Friedrich Engels in the nineteenth century. He was born in Trier in German and moved to London in 1849. He believed that societies are divided into two classes of people, those who own and control the structures and means of producing society's goods, the bourgeoisie, and those who own nothing or very little, the proletariat, who have to sell their labour to the first group to survive. Among the first group were the professions. While they were not owners of the means of production, they help to control its operation. The interests of these two groups – bourgeoisie and proletariat – are different and because of this society is characterized by class conflict. Marx understood the ownership of the means of production as the most important single variable in the history of human society. He saw human history in terms of a number of periods, or epochs, for example a period of early communism where people held everything in common. More recently a feudal society where wealth and production had been based on the land ownership of the aristocracy was replaced by the beginnings of today's capitalist society. Here technological development (for example Britain's 'industrial revolution' of the eighteenth and nineteenth centuries) has allowed the bourgeois class to exploit the efficiencies of factory-based production for its private gain. The aristocracy has either been sidelined or co-opted into the bourgeoisie. The only option for the majority of the people, however, is to become wage-labourers. Marx saw the West's colonization of great parts of the globe in terms of the ever more efficient exploitation of resources and labour. The main relations of production in this epoch are between employers and employees (to remind you,

---

5 There are many introductions to Marx and Marxism. One on-line resource is available from www.sociology.org.uk and at www.marxists.org. I have drawn on the latter in my summary here.

those who own and use capital and those who exchange their labour power for wages). Marx believed in an 'end of history' when the contradictions inherent in capitalism (that the means of production become owned by fewer and fewer people for example) would lead to its demise and the final epoch would be characterized by the ownership of the means of production by all, for the benefit of all.

Unlike other philosophers who Marx believed simply wished to interpret or understand the world, Marx's project was to change society and bring about the end of history – through revolution. The first stage of this project is to undertake a thorough critique of capitalist society in order to expose its workings. To that end he developed a number of arguments.

The first is about the operation of power. Those whose own and control the means of production are powerful in society because they can use their wealth to enhance and expand their power. However, this economically powerful class has to translate its power into i) political power in terms of control over the operation of government and ii) ideological power or control over how people think about the nature of the social world and their own place in it. Marx developed the notion of what we call hegemony, 'leadership with the consent of the led', to describe this. The ruling class can establish its hegemony over other classes through the use of force, for example through the police and by means of ideology and socialization via the mass media, the education system and the operation of social work for example. Marxist Louis Althusser, writing in 1970, called these forms of control 'ideological state apparatuses' (Althusser 1971).[6] Capitalist ideology makes other forms of organizing society literally unthinkable. The concept of false consciousness is a powerful one to explain how the proletariat is drawn in by

6 I talked in Chapter 6 about the UK mass media, noting that the majority of newspaper circulation is associated with a very small number of owners. The Leveson Inquiry, also mentioned in that chapter, showed this attempt to gain ideological power in action (Leveson The Right Honourable Lord Justice 2012).

the ruling class to the values of capitalist society, failing to see, according to Marx and followers of these ideas, their true position as members of an exploited and oppressed group.

Marx's second argument was that a 'total critique' of capitalism is needed to truly understand the operation of society and to understand that the way things appear is a result of a combination of economic, political and ideological conflicts. But understanding is the foundation for action. As he writes at the end of *The Communist Manifesto*, 'the proletarians have nothing to lose but their chains. They have a world to win' (Marx and Engels 1888 [1984] pp. 120–21).

Critiques of Marxism

You have already read that the Frankfurt School critical theorists were strongly influenced by the ideas of Marx but did not accept them uncritically – they were not called critical for nothing. There are a number of critiques of classic Marxism that you need to be aware of and I will spell these out below. Critiques come in many forms, some are theoretical and some are more 'common sense'. Let's start with the latter and move on to the former:

1   Marx, with his picture of a two-class society, did not foresee the enormous growth of what we call today, tellingly, the 'middle class', a class that probably includes you and me. It does not own the means of production but probably can be considered to be working to the benefit of those that do. It does, however, enjoy considerable economic advantages and, so far, stability. We are comfortable enough not to start a revolution. Globally there is a different picture and a far larger gulf between the wealth of the West and the so-called developing world. The rich countries clearly exploit the poor though there are perhaps growing middle classes within some of these countries – the apparently 'successful' emerging economies.

2   Marx's stages of history have not happened. Marx predicted that wages would fall and that capitalist economies would

suffer worsening economic crises that would lead to the overthrow of the capitalist system. The economic crises have clearly occurred but so far capitalism is proving resilient. He predicted that the most advanced economies would experience revolution first, however communist revolutions have occurred in poor countries, in parts of Latin America and, notably, in Russia in the early twentieth century.

3   Critics argue that the implementation of communism would lead not to a society run to the benefit of all but to despotic states. The power given to even former proletarian leaders would change their view of society leading them to no longer share the interests of the proletariat at large. The communist revolution in Russia (1917) clearly ushered in extreme totalitarian regimes and leaders as well as unfriendly hotel receptionists.

4   Marx claimed that his project was founded on science. Some claim that his 'laws' are vague or little more than philosophical dogma. Some critiques focus on the scientific claim itself arguing that Marx, as a creature of his time, looked to science as a strong form of authority, a way of claiming that his opponents were wrong. From that perspective, 'ideology' is the alternative to science. Many social scientists today would argue that science is simply another form of ideology.

5   Marx's view of the progress of history was influenced by German philosopher Friedrich Hegel (1770–1831). For Hegel it was 'spirit' that drove history forward. For Marx it was class conflict and proletarian consciousness. Critics question the possibility that history can be understood as 'progress' of any kind.

To end this summary of critiques I want to point out that on reading *The Communist Manifesto*, a short piece of fewer than 12,000 words written in 6 weeks in 1848, it is impossible not to be struck by its prophetic quality. The ever-increasing 'efficiency' of capitalism, increasing globalization, the concentration of the world's capital in fewer and fewer hands are stunningly contemporary.

What has Karl Marx ever done for us?[7]
Well, er . . .
Social Security
Pensions
Paid holidays
Trade Unions
Scholarships[8]
The idea of ideology and false consciousness
A rallying point for critiques of capitalism
The possibility of praxis: the enacting of a theory
The spectre

Other critiques: the Enlightenment and critique, Nietzsche and Foucault

Marx's ideas have been highly influential. They have provided concepts that cannot be put back in the box and a framework that is used by even those who disagree with his conclusions. But there are other flavours of critique that I want to mention before I end the chapter.

I hope it is not too unhelpfully general to understand critique as having historical origins in the questioning of or even the refusal to obey traditional forms of authority. The so-called Enlightenment (very approximately the late seventeenth and eighteenth centuries) in Europe is usually seen as a period of

---

7   For the reader who has no idea what this passage is about, I refer them to Monty Python's 1979 feature film *Life of Brian*. Reg, a parody of a working class revolutionary leader in Palestine at the time of Christ, played by John Cleese asks 'What have the Romans ever done for us?' His comrades effortlessly produce a list of things the Romans have done for us – drains to name just one. The film, in a tradition of British popular comedy, is replete with working class stereotypes: 'terrific race the Romans'.

8   This part of the list is taken from the cartoon book *Marx for Beginners*, (Rius 1994).

turning away from the dogmatic authority of the church. This took many forms: the Reformation was a movement that by making biblical scripture available to individual believers in their own language promised a faith without reliance on the official teachings of the Catholic church. Philosophers like Descartes and, later, Kant questioned in depth how the individual can gain knowledge and the processes of rational thought. Even questioning, sometimes dangerously, the rule of monarchs, philosophers critiqued the basis for their authority arguing that their rule needed to have a basis in rationality. Scepticism and questioning became driving forces in philosophical thought as critiques leapfrogged over one another. No sooner has science been proposed as promising emancipation from religion and superstition, than a critique of science as part of the armoury of state authority emerges. No sooner has the individual been placed centre stage than the individual is understood as a temporary phenomenon, a creation of governments in their efforts to control increasing populations.[9] No sooner has escape from ideology into truth been proposed than the notion of discourse emerges, a range of organized ways of understanding and speaking about the world that cannot be avoided.

The period laid the ground for the 'three masters of suspicion':[10] Marx, whom we have just discussed, Freud the psychoanalyst introduced in Chapters 1 and 2 who dared to propose that the individual, controlled by unconscious forces, was not 'master in his house', and Nietzsche (1844–1900). Friedrich Nietzsche was fiercely anti-religious. He proposed that the historical origin of Christianity's compassion for and identification with the 'meek' was little more than a fantasy of

---

9   I am thinking of the arguments of French historian Michel Foucault. He finds the origins of critique in the relationship of resistance to ecclesiastical authority. In relation to church doctrine, 'Not wanting to be governed was a certain way of refusing, challenging, limiting . . . ecclesiastical rule. It meant returning to the Scriptures . . .' and also 'Not to want to be governed. . . . Not wanting to accept these laws because they are unjust because . . . they hide a fundamental illegitimacy.'

10 The label is credited to philosopher Paul Ricoeur.

revenge against the powerful on the part of the powerless. He termed this a 'slave morality' and he clearly had a weak spot for the aristocratic 'beasts' who behaved as if they were above authority, like some kind of *Übermensch*, usually translated as 'superman'. Nursing's valuing of compassion has been likened to its 'slave morality', a fantasy of revenge on doctors. [11]

Where and how to find out more

If you are already familiar with the topics of this chapter you will realize that I have provided only a brief introduction. There is no shortage of books and on-line resources to be found if you want to study critical theory, or Marxism, or the work of the members of the Frankfurt School further. I suggest using on-line sources to gain an overview of the area and second hand book suppliers such as Abe Books to source the work of individual authors. There is nothing like holding a beautifully designed, though dog-eared, 1970s paperback in your hands. A useful and readable on-line resource is to be found at www.marxists.org and there are plenty of websites discussing the Frankfurt School in any amount of depth. It is better to investigate intensely than widely. And it is usually worth trying to read the words of authors themselves, albeit often in translation, rather than rely completely on books about them.

So, what does this mean for me?

Let's return to how this chapter started. I made the claim that if you look through the lenses of theory the world becomes a very different place from how it used to seem. Critical theory and perspectives informed by critical theory reveal the operation of power, often in the service of capital but also in the interests of particular groups such as powerful professions

---

11 This is in a paper by John Paley (2002) which is essential reading for anyone in nursing thinking seriously about critique. I have mentioned it before in this book.

and the class interests within them. Critical theory can bring some degree of empowerment because it gives you a framework to help make sense of experiences in healthcare and events in the news. After a while, thinking theoretically becomes a practice – it is how you are in the world, resilient because you are informed and no longer naïve. And the critical theorists were not content with analysis. They wanted to change society.

Chapter 9

Nursing solidarity, organizing and resistance

YASMIN (third-year Adult branch student): Well it depends how much you're immersed into the course though – some people will not be affected by it; they know how to switch it on and off, but I don't.

NILAM: Oh I can't switch it off.

YASMIN: I think it's a personality, like you are a nurse as a person, by the end of the course you are made into a different person; you haven't just gained knowledge –

NILAM: You are a nurse instead.

MICHAEL: That's interesting – can you say more?

NILAM: I am more protective about my family, for example, if I know that my family, they have some sort of illness, and I'm trying to analyse what's wrong with them and try to direct them to go to the GP or something, and it's not always working, but –

YASMIN: You don't switch off; you've always got your nursing head on once you become a nurse.

MICHAEL: What do you mean?

YASMIN: Like you're analytical, you're a bit more professional.

REEM: I feel like you're more human as well.

I want to end the main part of this book by discussing nursing solidarity, organizing for action and resistance. I will talk about how the rise of the Internet and social media have provided an arena and opportunity for nurses to organize, support each other and build networks.

Radical nurses past and present

Let's start by looking back a little. The Radical Nurses Group was set up in 1980 and was active for 10 years.[1] It described itself as 'a way of getting together, to support each other, to help us feel we're not alone, to moan together perhaps, to discuss our common problems but also hopefully to act together to change things'. It was ambitious in its intentions:

> Staff shortages, sex roles and stereotyping in nursing, nurses, trade unionism and militancy, nurses roles, especially in relation to doctors, lack of emotional support for nurses and many others – the problem is which to tackle first!
> (Confederation of Health Service Employees [COHSE] 2006)

Among other topics it grappled with the place of a pre-dominantly female profession in the male dominated trade union movement and put the term 'professional organizations' in inverted commas, presumably to distance itself from what it saw as the RCN's conservatism. From today's perspective many nurses would be surprised that the group gave so much attention to the problems with and challenge of working with and alongside the medical profession. Perhaps the class and gender inequalities between nurses and doctors were stronger in the 1980s than they are now or perhaps a new, at least perceived, challenge to professional nursing has emerged in the shape of managerialist interventions at the behest of governments. The group 'refused to cope'. They made a badge with this slogan. They meant, I believe, that nursing did not do itself – or healthcare – any favours by grudgingly putting up with a series of cuts and indignities, complaining but never taking action. The slogan on their badge reminds me of a piece in a book about photography, written by critic John Berger, about an image of

---

1   Many thanks to the grumbling appendix for her archive and discussion of the RNG at www.newleftproject.org. I draw on her observations in this section.

the dead Cuban revolutionary Che Guevara taken in 1967. Guevara was well aware that his stance and his actions might well lead to his death and he put in writing the fact that he had no reservations about this. He fought, to put it very simply, against injustice and exploitation and knew how strong their forces were. Berger writes: 'His envisaged death offered him the measure of how intolerable his life would be if he accepted the intolerable condition of the world as it is' (Berger 2013 p. 8). This word 'intolerable' is repeated throughout the chapter on Che and others who have given their lives for their beliefs about injustice. Later Berger writes, 'The world is not intolerable until the possibility of transforming it exists but is denied.' In contrast to the world's poor, nurses in the UK are privileged. However, as people who deal, sometimes on a daily basis, with extremes of suffering and death, it does not seem not far-fetched to sometimes see the conditions that others expect them to do this work within as exploitative, exploitative of their urge to help others for example. I cannot help but see the suggestion that nurses cope better and learn how to be more resilient as, wittingly or not, a part of that exploitation. That is why that small badge offers so much power. What is intolerable should be named as such not put up with.

The Radical Nurses Group held national meetings in London, Sheffield and Manchester, formed regional groups and planned local level events. Those who wanted to keep in touch with the group were asked to send six stamped addressed envelopes and £1 to receive a regular newsletter for the year.[2] However, unlike the 1980s, today nurses do not need to get on a train to find a venue to meet or lick stamps to keep up to date. Even when events are unfolding quickly, such as the student protests against the new tuition fees in 2010, a distributed and instant platform like Twitter enabled those on the front line of the protest to tell

---

2   The rise of the printed newsletter was aided by the increasing use of personal computers, particularly desktop publishing on the Apple Macintosh. The late 1980s and the 1990s was a period of radical and subversive typography.

many hundreds of others what is happening. Activism is easier now. Today the #BursaryOrBust hashtag is being used by a student group to share information about the government plan to replace the student nurse bursary with a loan on which interest is payable, to organize protests, spread their counter-arguments and to make links with other radical groups. One advantage that spontaneously formed groups have over more formal bodies like the RCN is that they can make decisions and act more quickly, and because they are a small group brought together by a single issue about which its members are likely to be in agreement. The RCN may have more than 420,000 members but the vast majority do not take the opportunity to vote when there is a ballot for industrial action.[3] And on any given issue there are likely to be large groups holding contradictory views. This can reflect the personal politics of individual members or where they are placed in the health and education industries, reflecting sectional interests. For example on the question of degree-level entry to the profession, a nurse educator and a nurse manager may well have different opinions because they have different priorities. Nevertheless these large bodies like the RCN, other healthcare and public sector unions and the British Medical Association (BMA) are able to speak for and stand up for the profession they represent. It is to their achievements and the problems they face that I will now turn.

Nursing unions and their achievements

Solidarity is the historical basis of the union movement. The first step of those promoting union membership is to convince workers that only in unity will they gain the means to change their existence. Those who employ workers, whether they are nineteenth-century factory owners or today's large corporations,

3 Former General Secretary Peter Carter told me that when the government planned to introduce changes to the NHS pension scheme that would affect nurses, the RCN balloted its members for action. Only 16% voted and of those, 40% voted to accept the new, less attractive, proposal.

have the advantage that they are already organized and can set terms and conditions to which each individual employee has to agree if they want the work. For public sector workers like nurses, the employer that they have to deal with is the government itself. Control of the NHS has been a thorn in the side of governments almost since it was created. I have set out some of the detail in Chapter 6. Governments have progressively set up mechanisms and bodies to measure so-called efficiency, productivity and quality within the service and an increasing set of incentives and punishments for managers of NHS organizations to achieve various targets, creating pressures that are passed down to the individual nurse in the clinic or on the ward.

Organizations like the RCN and the British Medical Association (BMA) have a contradictory, or at least a difficult role with governments. As professional organizations they have to maintain good relationships with civil servants and ministers to contribute to government health policies. But as trade unions representing the interests of their members they have to enter into possibly confrontational encounters. One of the roles that a union plays is to support its members to take industrial action by withdrawing their labour. At the time of writing the Junior Doctors Committee of the BMA is locked in conflict with the Department of Health over pay for unsocial hours with junior doctors striking on a number of occasions. The same issue, raised in 2015, caused the RCN alongside other unions Unite and UNISON to threaten strike action (Cooper and McSmith 2015).

The RCN has not always been so supportive of strike action. It was only in 1995 that it decided to amend its 'Rule 12' to allow the RCN to authorize the possibility of strike action by nurses as long as such action was not considered 'detrimental to the well-being or interests of their patients or clients'. Before this its refusal to permit its members to strike was sometimes a cause of controversy. By the RCN itself and, possibly, governments of the day, it was seen a sign of its responsibility and professionalism. It was, after all, given a place on various pay determining bodies. But by members of other unions and by more militantly minded members it was seen as a failure to take its trade union identity seriously and as a lack of solidarity with other healthcare workers.

There is, as yet, no legal constraint on nurses taking strike action and the NMC Code does not prevent nurses and midwives from taking part in lawful industrial action however, the RCN has never called for industrial action or a strike.

Social media and activism

The growth of platforms such as Facebook, Twitter and YouTube, coupled with mobile technology that enables connection to the Internet from almost any location have made it possible for individuals to continually post data on-line. The trouble is that most of what is posted tends to be banal and likely to be of interest, apart from to the person who posted it, only to historians of culture from the distant future or curious observers from other planets. Social media is also used by individuals, sometimes prominent, who forget that their bigotry, bullying or boasting – or just unguarded humour – is visible to the whole world. Some high-profile resignations started with a comment on Facebook or Twitter. Some who identify themselves as professionals in their posts have used social media as the platform for a kind of talk that is usually considered 'back room' (see my discussion in Chapter 4 of Daniel Chambliss' observations on nurses talking about traumatic events), sometimes identifying co-workers or patients in the process. The profession and individual employers are clearly anxious about this potential blot on their reputations. The RCN has issued what it has called legal advice for members about Internet usage and the NMC also provide guidance on the use of social media by nurses on their website.[4] The relevance of social media to this book, however, is its use for political activism and networking and this is already well-established.

4   At the time of writing this is available at www.rcn.org.uk/__data/assets/ pdf_file/0008/272195/003557.pdf. The NMC's guidance is currently at www.nmc-uk.org/Nurses-and-midwives/Regulation-in-practice/Regulation-in-Practice-Topics/Social-networking-sites/

The rise of demonstrations across the Arab world between 2010 and 2012, known as the 'Arab Spring' was well reported as being enabled by the use of social media. Using social media and smart phones enabled protesters both to rapidly spread information to organize and to transmit video shot on phones across the world to mobilize sympathies for their causes (Lindsey 2013).[5] The regimes under threat in some of these countries attempted to block access to these media,[6] giving an idea of their perceived power.

In the UK there are many campaigning groups and intelligent Internet interventions by nurses commenting on NHS policy and seeking change. Because the Internet can change so quickly it is difficult to recommend any particular website. There are a great many blogs written by nurses. Many offer informal reflection on the work of a nurse in particular settings and it is hard to delineate those which could be considered as activism from those which are either personal observations or sharing of clinical information – important as these are. At the time of writing, I recommend these examples of Internet sites and social media developed by nurses to do what they do best which is to create an arena for honest debate and to move opinion and information around a network.

- One nursing blog that is gaining followers and attention is *the grumbling appendix* (https://grumblingappendix.word press.com/about/). Its mysterious author writes sometimes with withering satire about nursing in the NHS, focussing on managerial and government-induced absurdities. When most public figures in nursing and the NHS go to great lengths to present a bad situation in a positive light, the grumbling appendix offers blistering critique with satirical humour. Comments from readers are also well-written and insightful.

5   For a collection of analyses of the role of social media in the Arab uprisings see: www.westminster.ac.uk/__data/assets/pdf_file/0004/220675/WPCC-vol9-issue2.pdf

6   See http://en.wikipedia.org/wiki/Internet_censorship_in_the_Arab_Spring

- Jane Salvage (www.janesalvage.com). Jane was one of the original founders of the Radical Nurses Group and is still a policy activist. Her website and blog acts as a repository of her writing, for example national newspaper articles about all degree nurse education.
- Nurse Manifest is a blog set up by a collective of North American nurse activists in 2000 and still going strong. The site includes a lengthy manifesto of the beliefs of the group and findings of research it carried out into the working lives of nurses. https://nursemanifest.com/
- Centre for Critical Research in Nursing & Midwifery http://critresnurse.org. This is the unit where I work. We have been developing 'Critical Briefings' on current health service and nursing news designed as pdf documents to download, print and wave around. The site also houses a blog and is linked to the centre's Twitter feed.

Finally a word of warning: alongside blogs and social media creations that are the work of real people, many corporations and institutions have, of course, launched their own, not wanting to be left behind. Often their fundamental aim is self-promotion and attracting market share. Many blogs with 'nurse' in the title turn out to be of this kind, perhaps written by university or NHS media departments or recruitment agencies or sponsored by publishers. They can be a useful source of knowledge but they are unlikely to have the vitality, wit, criticality or honesty of the best individual work.

Benefits and risks

Many commentators have written about the benefits and the risks of the rapid development of a radically connected society that the Internet, social media and smart phones have made possible (Van Dijck 2013). Much of the 'digital risk' is to do with the impact on privacy and the rise in possibilities for surveillance (Beck 2013). Those who are critical of the rise of a 'surveillance society' warn that users of these technologies wittingly or unwittingly make intimate aspects of their lives available for retrieval and scrutiny by corporations who wish to target us with their products and services, by governments who wish to monitor their population's activities for reasons of national security, political advantage or paranoia, and by employers and potential employers who wish to assess the profile of employees or job candidates (Allan *et al.* 2016). In other words, social media is to be used with caution.

> There is something paradoxical about the Internet and social media. Computers and smart phones deal with fleeting and impermanent movements of electricity. Connections arise and pass. Turn them off and everything in their memory evaporates. But what gets said on the Internet is resilient and sticks around, probably for ever, for far longer than you can remember what you said.

Nurses of all countries unite: no nurse need be alone

The main message of this book is a call to move away from an individualistic understanding of healthcare, nursing work and resilience. The tendency to think in terms of the individual rather than of communities has been a characteristic of Western societies since, perhaps, the time of the Enlightenment that I talked about in the previous chapter. It has been drawn upon and exploited by neoliberal governments in the UK and US for the last 25 years and is at work in many policies that affect nursing. The end of student bursaries is not only a shifting of the cost of nurse education from the Department of Health to the individual student, but a shift in principle. The measurement of quality and productivity in healthcare, and in universities, is carried out at lower and lower levels even though any individual nurse or unit's so-called performance is influenced by structural forces far beyond their control. Everywhere there are forces that divide us. From all directions we face the imperative to take individual responsibility for our actions and even our feelings within constraints that we did not choose and that we do not support. If we stumble it is noted and we are asked to account for ourselves, asked what help we need. To acquiesce to the demand of resilience is to agree to take responsibility for a situation for which others are responsible. It is to let others off the hook. Nursing and healthcare work is perhaps uniquely traumatic but the conditions within which the work is done are a result of actual decisions taken by men and women in a site far from the work itself. When the individual nurse's consciousness is so shaped that she fails to understand this, beyond a general complaint about being uncared for by governments, then the work of neoliberalism is perfected.

Social media enables nurses to overcome these individualizing, or 'responsibilizing' forces. It allows us to develop conversations and networks irrespective of where we are and what time of the day or night it is. Because of this the idea of community and our possibilities for support and solidarity are massively expanded. Social media offers opportunities for increased democracy and voice. Although those with power, whether governments or large corporations, take up significant space on the Internet in addition to their influence via conventional media such as national newspapers and television channels, many critical voices are now able to gain audiences in ways that were almost impossible in earlier times. Evidence of corruption or corporate dishonesty, for example, can be instantly presented to a global audience. Critiques and alternative views can be more easily expressed.

Being a student nurse is not a position that holds a great deal of power either in the National Health Service or within the profession itself, but today, no student, nor registered nurse, need be alone and unconnected. In Chapter 2 I suggested that getting together and getting informed are the first steps in developing critical resilience. In this chapter I have presented some models of what can result when nurses organize.

Survive and act to change.

Nurses have nothing to lose but their chains. They have a world to win.

Appendix

Summary of the research papers on resilience in nursing in this book

The search was carried out via EBSCOhost in July 2015 of the CINHAL database. The keywords used were nurs* and resilien*. Only peer-reviewed research articles written in the English language were included and related words were included. The search brought up 278 articles. After the search was run articles without direct relevance to nurses and nursing practice were discarded. Full references to articles are given in the reference list. The following represents my notes on the found articles.

Ablett 2007 explores 'personality constructs of hardiness and sense of coherence'. The research is framed as within a salutogenic paradigm i.e. with an intention to focus on the factors that might explain why some individuals remain healthy under conditions of stress. Ten interviews of qualitative research of nurses in palliative care. Resilience encapsulated by personality traits – hardiness and 'sense of coherence' which are described as 'protective factors'. No organizational factors included in this analysis so it departs from the classic approach in resilience research with children. Also study carried out in a single setting so no way of identifying if any outcomes are related to characteristics of the setting. Concludes that staff training could be used to develop both these personality factors.

Cameron and Brownlee 2010, qualitative with nine nurses in aged care setting. All reference to 'resilience' is from nursing literature. Study carried out in a single setting so no way of identifying if any outcomes are related to characteristics of the setting. Resilience understood as a set of skills that can be learned that can help coping. Assumption that nurses who remain in difficult clinical settings in general must have some positive characteristics and do not stay as a result of what might be considered negative such as lack of alternative employment, lack of confidence to move into other settings. Motivation seen as protective. Circularity evident: nurses were encouraged to reflect on the following statement: 'Resilience is the ability to rebound from adversity and overcome difficult circumstances in one's life.' Participants appear to identify factors that promote job satisfaction but label these 'resilience'.

Jacelon 1997 review of resilience 'as trait and process'. Appears to lack some of the nuances of the best resilience studies, focussing on 'a trait inherent in individuals' or 'a process which one may be able to learn' (p. 123). Reviews some studies of 'resilience' among adults. Some (Wagnild and Young 1990) seem particularly circular i.e. resilient people are found to be persevering, self-reliant, etc. Research on resilience in adults seems to focus on personality traits and take less notice of community-based influences than studies of children and adolescents. The review concludes with some weak recommendations that are designed to help nurses recognize and foster resilience in their patients before illness and after crises.

Dolan *et al.* 2012 study of 16 haemodialysis nurses in one hospital and two of its satellite units. Lower levels of burnout said to suggest increased resilience among this speciality therefore an apparent 'need to better understand how haemodialysis nurses perceive and cope with stressors in a way that reduces burnout and promotes resilience' (p. 223). No details of recruitment or of size of population of nurses or comparison of presumed volunteers to the others. Recruitment stopped when data was saturated. Same sample completed measures of burnout and of resilience. Qualitative findings focus on specific probably atypical themes of blurred boundaries and conflict between young and old nurses. Data is under-analysed. Supposed fundamental delineation between emotional distancing and depersonalization or negative attitudes to patients on a few specific and short quotations. No references to resilience literature.

Manzano García and Ayala Calvo's brief definitions of resilience (2012). Sample of 200 completed measures including the Connor–Davidson Resilience Scale (CD-RISC) (Connor and Davidson 2003). Of the 25 items in this scale, 15 were removed from the authors' explanatory model. One part of the understanding of the resilience literature is the suggestion made by some that adversity may be a necessary part of development in order to develop some aspects of resilience. Manzano García and colleagues recommend staff training to developing coping skills but they observe paradoxically: 'However, it is important to acknowledge that work stress and crises are inevitable and even necessary for the growth and maturity of the individual and to allow them to reach their full potential' (p. 105).

Gillespie *et al*. 2007. Survey of 1430 operating room nurses investigates 'resilience' in terms of its correlation with five psychological variables (hope, self-efficacy, coping, control and competence). It concludes that educational programmes for nurses could focus on identifying nurses 'at risk', developing these characteristics in order to increase resilience and 'and thus retain nurses in this specialty' (p. 427). No attention to work processes or the organizational or professional environment and all the 'variables', including those that refer to external events such as collaboration are assessed by asking the individuals to rate their view of these rather than by any external assessment of these.

Jackson *et al*. 2007. Review of 'personal resilience' as a 'strategy for surviving'. Again assumes that nurses who 'remain in nursing' have chosen to do this, with the assumption of individuals as free actors in a market for work. Understands 'resilience' as 'the ability of an individual to positively adjust to adversity . . .' and that 'nurses can actively participate in the development and strengthening of their own personal resilience to reduce their vulnerability to workplace adversity and thus improve the overall healthcare setting' (p. 1), however in their introduction to the 'adversity' of the workplace, the factors are all external workforce issues, casualization, staff shortages, bullying, abuse and violence. Naïve assumption based on an understanding of resilience in terms of personal skills 'If equilibrium is maintained, an individual can theoretically manage any situation that comes along. Thus, we argue that developing personal resilience can reduce vulnerability' (p. 3).

Some researchers (Hodges *et al.* 2008) recommend that student nurses are taught 'strategies of reflective learning and reflexive practice' (p. 4) and argue 'that resilience can be developed and may help retain nurses in the profession, rather than abandoning their career path when the complexities of providing health care seem overwhelming' (p. 5). Exaggerated views 'Protective factors help individuals to achieve a positive outcome regardless of the risk' (p. 5). Claim that 'positive emotions' and 'optimism' can buffer against life adversity. The recommendations are superficial and naïve amounting to little more than the injunction to 'think positively!' Develop insight into your own emotions, learn to laugh and to take up physical activities outside work but developing insight into the causes of the workplace adversity or joining with others to effect change is ignored.

Larrabee *et al.* 2010. The initial problem is nurse turnover in the US: 'Turnover cost per nurse ranged from $62,000 to $67,000 in a recent study (Jones 2005), and results of another study (Waldman *et al.* 2004) indicated that the annual nurse turnover cost for an academic medical centre ranged from 3.4% to 5.8% of the organization's budget (Larrabee *et al.* 2010 p. 82). Many work environment factors lead to job satisfaction and dissatisfaction. One of the other possible causes is 'psychological empowerment'. Recommendations: Include training interventions aimed at increasing 'psychological empowerment': The goal of primary interventions would be to 'eliminate or reduce job stressors' (p. 223) and would be aimed at making changes in the organization. The goal of secondary interventions would be to 'alter the ways that individuals perceive or respond to stressors' and would be aimed at individuals (p. 223), as would the proposed psychological empowerment training programmes. Finally, the goal of tertiary interventions would be to treat individuals with job stress–related illness to help them recover and return to work (p. 96).

Koen *et al.* 2011. Large quantitative study comparing 'resilience' of nurses in public and private organizations. Some of the usual assumptions: 'although many nurses consider leaving the profession, some resiliently survive, cope and even thrive despite the workplace adversity experienced' (p. 1). The context is South Africa's recently changed public healthcare system where a restructuring has placed an enormous burden on healthcare workers in this part of the system, involving a serious shortage of nurses leading to a ratio of 468 patients for 1 nurse. The nation has a sharply divided health system so that the private part is better resourced. In this context the author looks hopefully to positive psychology to shore up what appears to be a healthcare system in a state of considerable dysfunction and crisis: 'Resilience has become an appealing concept because of its roots in theoretical models of positive psychology that seek to explore factors that enable individuals to successfully overcome adversity' (p. 2). The so-called characteristics of 'resilient people' echoes the popular fascination with the practices of 'successful people'. We have moved a long way from the warnings of the leaders in the field of resilience research not to consider resilience simply as an individual's inner quality but to associate resilience with systems/contexts and the individual's response to these. In the face of appalling health need and inadequacy of the system, the author focuses on the need for nurses to show effective coping behaviours, a 'sense of coherence', optimism and hope. The author claims that understanding resilience among nurses 'would provide hospital managers with useful guidelines for in-service training that won't be threatening and can facilitate growth in professional nurses' (p. 3). This hope seems to be based on a probably realistic pessimism that nurses are able to influence the system as a whole in that country. Findings were that nurses in the private sector reported higher emotional well-being and resilience. This suggests to me that what is being discussed here as 'resilience' is a response to context and that the author's discussion of 'resilient people' does not fit with these findings.

Matos *et al.* 2010. Small US quantitative study with same intention: to understand resilience and job satisfaction in order to implement nurse retention programmes specifically targeted toward teaching nurses skills in developing resilience. Claim for particularity for mental health nursing. 'By definition, a resilient individual is able to prevail in the face of stress, and resilient nurses could be well suited for work in the mental health environment' (Matos *et al.* 2010 p. 308). Survey of 32 nurses, total number of staff is not given nor are any details of sampling or recruitment. This is a small sample compared with other quantitative studies. Wagnild and Young measure used to measure 'resilience which the authors defined as a positive personality characteristic that enhances individual adaptation' (p. 309). Again the concept is used separately from any understanding of resilience as a dynamic between the individual and their environment. Only two non-nursing journal references.

Maxwell *et al.* (2011). Qualitative interview study with 10 nurses, looking at the transition to qualification, trying to draw on an understanding of resilience that 'shifts the emphasis from resilience as an individual trait or acquired skill to a more interactional definition, incorporating wider social, cultural and organizational factors' (p. 428). The paper makes little contribution to the study of resilience and is largely descriptive and atheoretical.

McDonald *et al.* (2012). Report of an intervention with 14 nurses and midwives designed to develop 'personal resilience'. The scene is set by a listing of workplace factors creating 'adversity' and the key argument for turning to individual factors is:

> Undoubtedly there is a need to improve organizational approaches to workplace adversity and the systemic environmental problems that persist in the nursing and midwifery workplace. Nonetheless, there is a continuing need to promote personal responses that emphasize positive ways to support and learn from each other about surviving and thriving in nursing and midwifery.
>
> (McDonald *et al.* 2012 p. 378)

Participants selected from particularly adverse wards. The aims are highly individualized: 'A principal aim of the intervention model was to facilitate positive responses to the participants' workplace environment through the exploration of practical and relevant coping strategies. The underlying premise was that greater insight and understanding of the self – "a person's view of her own unique being" (Porritt 1990 p. 47) – could improve individual performance (p. 379). Content was based on a review of what have been considered the components of resilience. Evaluation in the form of 'Evaluative comments from participants were collected from postintervention interviews, workshop evaluations, field notes and a research journal completed after each workshop' (p. 382). No pre and post 'measurement' of resilience. The evaluation was carried out by the team who also devised and delivered the intervention. The experience was clearly very satisfying and engaging.

Mealer *et al.* (2012). A national US survey of 744 intensive care nurses using the Connor–Davidson Resilience Scale alongside measures of psychological disorders including burnout and post-traumatic stress disorder, showed a correlation. Those rated to have high resilience had lower scores on the psychological disorders. The rationale is a global nurse shortage particularly in the specialist area of ICU and nurses leaving the profession because of workplace dissatisfaction. The survey showed high amounts of burnout and post-traumatic stress disorder (PTSD) among their sample. They conclude 'Because resilience can be learned, educational programmes for ICU nurses may result in fewer distress symptoms, improved job satisfaction, and potentially decrease the high turnover rate for ICU nurses' (Mealer *et al.* 2012 p. 297). Ten psychological characteristics can be learned to help increase resilience, including: optimism, developing cognitive flexibility, developing a personal moral compass or set of beliefs, altruism, finding a resilient role-model or mentor, learning to be adept at facing fear, developing active coping skills, having a supportive social network, exercising, and having a sense of humour (p. 297). Resilience training, they conclude, could lead to nurses who will 'thrive at the bedside for extended periods of time' and could also identify nurses with low resilience who can be targeted with interventions.

Mealer *et al.* (2012). Qualitative companion piece to the above article with telephone interviews with 27 nurses in two groups – those with high resilience and those with high PTSD scores. Same argument: nursing shortage due to poor retention due to poor job satisfaction due to stress in ICU. The authors analysed the data and produced four themes that they believe characterize the highly scoring resilient nurses. Their dichotomous comparisons between the two groups are not necessarily rigorous and the quantitative comparisons between the percentages that mentioned various topics, e.g. spirituality, are questionable.

Zander *et al.* (2010). Literature review of 'coping and its relationship to resilience' looking for applicability in paediatric oncology nursing. Repeats the claim by Jackson *et al.* (2007) that 'there is a clear need for nurses to develop resilience to positively overcome the professional obstacles the health care system and workplace pose on them' (Zander *et al.* 2010 p. 95).

References

Ablett, J. R. and R. S. Jones (2007). "Resilience and well-being in palliative care staff: a qualitative study of hospice nurses' experience of work." *Psycho-Oncology* **16**(8): 733-740.

Allan, H., H. Cowie and P. Smith (2009). "Overseas nurses' experiences of discrimination: a case of racist bullying." *Journal of Nursing Management* **17**: 898–906.

Allan, H., M. Traynor, D. Kelly and P. Smith (2016). "Becoming a nurse." *Understanding Sociology in Nursing*. London, Sage: 50–70.

Althusser, L. (1971). *For Marx*. London, Allen Lane.

Anthony, E. J. and B. J. Cohler, eds (1987). *The Invulnerable Child*. The Guilford Psychiatry Series. New York, The Guilford Press.

Ashforth, B. E. and R. H. Humphrey (1993). "Emotional labor in service roles: The influence of identity." *The Academy of Management Review* **18**(1): 88–115.

Audit Commission (1996). *Fundholding facts: A digest of information about practices within the scheme during the first five years*. London, HMSO.

Baly, M. (1995). *Nursing and Social Change*. London, Routledge.

Batty, D. (6 December 2007). "Serial killer nurse Allitt must serve 30 years." Retrieved 10 October 2014, from www.theguardian.com/uk/2007/dec/06/ukcrime.health

BBC Panorama. (2011). "Undercover care: The abuse exposed." Retrieved 9 June 2011, from ww.bbc.co.uk/programmes/b011pwt6

Beck, U. (2013). "The digital freedom risk: too fragile an acknowledgement." *OpenDemocracy*. Retrieved 22 November 2014, from www.opendemocracy.net/can-europe-make-it/ulrich-beck/digital-freedom-risk-too-fragile-acknowledgment

Becker, H. S., B. Geer, E. C. Hughes and A. L. Strauss (1961). *Boys in White: Student Culture in Medical School*. Chicago, IL, University of Chicago Press.

Benner, P., C. A. Tanner and C. Chesla (1996). *Expertise in Nursing Practice. Caring, Clinical Judgement and Ethics*. New York, Springer.

Benner, P. and J. Wrubel (1989). *The Primacy of Caring: Stress and Coping in Health and Illness*. Boston MA, Addison-Wesley.

Berger, J. (2013). *Understanding a Photograph*. London, Penguin.

Berridge, V. (2006). "The policy response to the smoking and lung cancer connection in the 1950s and 1960s." *Historical Journal (Cambridge, England)* 49(4): 1185–1209.

Bhardwa, S. (2016). "Senior nurses condemn the closure of the DH nursing unit." Retrieved 6 July 2016, from www.independentnurse. co.uk/news/senior-nurses-condemn-the-closure-of-the-dh-nursing-unit/142310/

Bikker, A. P., B. Fitzpatrick, D. Murphy and S. W. Mercer (2015). "Measuring empathic, person-centred communication in primary care nurses: Validity and reliability of the Consultation and Relational Empathy (CARE) Measure." *BMC Family Practice* 16(149): 1–9.

Brindle, D. (17 March 1995). Minister says £120m surplus is evidence of fundholding success. *The Guardian*. London.

Broomfield, M. (20 March 2016). "Budget 2016: George Osborne cuts £1.1bn from NHS repairs fund." *UK Politics*. Retrieved 3 August 2016, from www.independent.co.uk/news/uk/politics/budget-2016-george-osborne-cuts-11bn-from-nhs-repairs-fund-a6942301.html

Buchan, J. (1993). "Matching supply with demand for nurses." *Nursing Standard* 7(46): 39.

Buchan, J. (2013). "The NHS workforce: how do we balance cost-effectiveness with safety?" *Time to Think Differently*. Retrieved 22 July 2014, from www.kingsfund.org.uk/time-to-think-differently/blog/nhs-workforce-balance-cost-effectiveness-safety

Buchanan, D., D. Denyer, J. Jaina, C. Kelliher, C. Moore, E. Parry and C. Pilbeam (2013). "How do they manage? A qualitative study of the realities of middle and front-line management work in health care." *Health Services and Delivery Research*, National Institute for Health Research, No. 1.4.

Buresh, B. and S. Gordon (2006). *From Silence to Voice: What Nurses Know and Must Communicate to the Public*. Ithaca, NY, ILR Press.

Buse, K., N. Mays and G. Walt (2005). *Making Health Policy*. Berkshire, UK, Open University Press.

Cameron, F. and S. Brownie (2010). "Enhancing resilience in registered aged care nurses." *Australasian Journal on Ageing* 29(2): 66–71.

Cartwright, S. and C. L. Cooper (2007). "Hazards to health: The problem of workplace bullying." *The Psychologist*. Retrieved 20 March 2016, from https://thepsychologist.bps.org.uk/volume-20/edition-5/hazards-health-problem-workplace-bullying

Cavendish, C. (2013). *The Cavendish Review: An Independent Review into Healthcare Assistants and Support Workers in the NHS and Social Care Settings*. London, Department of Health.

Chambliss, D. F. (1996). *Beyond Caring, Hospitals, Nurses and the Social Organization of Ethics*. Chicago, IL, Chicago University Press.

Chicago Women's Liberation Union (1970). "Consciousness-raising by the Women's Collective (Archive)." Retrieved 1 December 2015, from www.uic.edu/orgs/cwluherstory/CWLUArchive/crguidelines.html

Chief Nursing Officer for England and National Quality Board (2014). *How to Ensure the Right People, with the Right Skills, Are in the Right Place at the Right Time: A Guide to Nursing, Midwifery and Care Staffing Capacity And Capability*. London, National Quality Board.

Clarke, S. (2005). "The neoliberal theory of society." Retrieved 22 July 2016, from http://homepages.warwick.ac.uk/~syrbe/pubs/Neoliberalism.pdf

Collinson, P. (28 May 2016). "Student loans: The next big mis-selling scandal?" Retrieved 2 August , 2016, from www.theguardian.com/money/blog/2016/may/28/student-loans-next-mis-selling-scandal

Commissioning Board Chief Nursing Officer and DH Chief Nursing Adviser (2012). *Compassion in Practice: Nursing, Midwifery and Care Staff Our Vision and Strategy*. London, Department of Health NHS Commissioning Board.

Confederation of Health Service Employees (COHSE). (2006, September, 2006). "Radical nurses group." Retrieved 19 July 2016, from http://cohse-union.blogspot.co.uk/2006/09/radical-nurses-group-estb-1980.html

Conlon, G. and R. Ladher (2016). *The Impact of the 2015 Comprehensive Spending Review on Higher Education Fees and Funding Arrangements in Subjects Allied to Medicine*. London, London Economics.

Connor, K. M. and J. R. T. Davidson (2003). "Development of a new resilience scale: the Connor-Davidson resilience scale (CD-RISC)." *Depression and Anxiety* 18: 76–82.

Cooper, C. (2015). "NHS warning over hospitals 'fiddling figures' to meet targets." Retrieved 28 July 2016, from www.independent.co.uk/life-style/health-and-families/health-news/healthcare-experts-accuse-nhs-of-fiddling-figures-to-meet-performance-targets-10193482.html

Cooper, C. and A. McSmith (18 May 2015). "Nurses may call strike if government tries to cut pay as David Cameron vows to deliver 'truly seven-day NHS' plans." Retrieved 2 September 2015, from www.independent.co.uk/life-style/health-and-families/health-news/nursesmay-call-strike-over-plans-for-truly-sevenday-nhs-10256874.html

Curtis, K., K. Horton and P. Smith (2012). "Student nurse socialisation in compassionate practice: A Grounded Theory study." *Nurse Education Today* 32(7): 790–95.

Darbyshire, P. (2014). "Character assassination? Response to John Paley, 'Social psychology and the compassion deficit'." *Nurse Education Today* 34(6): 887–89.

De Saussure, F. (1996). Selections from the course in general linguistics. *The Continental Philosophy Reader*. R. Kearney and M. Rainwater (eds). London, Routledge: 291–304.

Department of Business, Innovation and Skills (2015). *Fulfilling Our Potential: Teaching Excellence, Social Mobility and Student Choice*. London, I. a. S. Business.

Department of Health (1989). *Working for Patients*. London, HMSO, Cmd 555.

Department of Health (1997). *The New NHS; Modern Dependable*. London, Department of Health, Cm. 3807.

Department of Health (1999). *Making a Difference, Strengthening the Nursing, Midwifery and Health Visiting Contribution to Health and Healthcare*. London, Department of Health.

Department of Health (2000). *The NHS Plan: A Plan for Investment, a Plan for Reform*. London, Department of Health.

Department of Health (2013). *Delivering High Quality, Effective, Compassionate Care: Developing the Right People with the Right Skills and the Right Values*. London, Department of Health.

Department of Health (9 December 2015). "NHS Bursary Reform: Changes to healthcare education funding for student nursing, midwifery and allied health students." (Updated 7 April 2016). Retrieved 1 August 2016, from www.gov.uk/government/publications/nhs-bursary-reform

Derrida, J. (1982). "Différance." *Margins of Philosophy*. Hemel Hempstead, UK, Harvester Wheatsheaf: 1–27.

Dinkins, C. (10 May 2011). "Ethics: Beyond Patient Care: Practicing Empathy in the Workplace." *OJIN: The Online Journal of Issues in Nursing*. Retrieved 24 January 2016, from www.nursingworld.org/MainMenuCategories/ANAMarketplace/ANAPeriodicals/OJIN/Columns/Ethics/Empathy-in-the-Workplace.html

Dixon, J. (2008). "Editorial." *British Medical Journal* 336: 844–45.

Dolan, G., E. Strodl and E. Hamernik (2012). "Why renal nurses cope so well with their workplace stressors." *Journal of Renal Care* 38(4): 222–32.

Dowling, E. (2007). "Producing the dining experience: Measure, subjectivity and the affective worker." *Ephemera* 7(1): 117–32.

Dunn, P. (2016). "What has the impact been of recent caps on NHS agency staff spend?" *Kings Fund Blog*. Retrieved 2 August 2016, from www.kingsfund.org.uk/blog/2016/03/nhs-agency-staff-spend 2016

Earvolino-Ramirez, M. (2007). "Resilience: A concept analysis." *Nursing Forum* 42(2): 73–82.

Fealy, G. M. (2004). " 'The good nurse': Visions and values in images of the nurse." *Journal of Advanced Nursing* 46(6): 649–56.

Fearon, C. and M. Nicol (2011). "Strategies to assist prevention of burnout in nursing staff." *Nursing Standard* 26(14): 35–9.

Ford, S. (2012). "Review concludes NMC is failing 'at every level'." Retrieved 16 August 2012, from www.nursingtimes.net/nursing-practice/clinical-specialisms/management/review-concludes-nmc-is-failing-at-every-level/5046648.article

Ford, S. (12 November 2013). "RCN warns of hidden crisis, as 20,000 nursing posts are unfilled." Retrieved 3 August, 2016, from www.nursingtimes.net/roles/nurse-managers/rcn-warns-of-hidden-crisis-as-20000-nursing-posts-are-unfilled/5065205.fullarticle

Foucault, M. (1997). "What is critique?" *What is Enlightenment? Eighteenth-Century Questions and Twentieth Century Answers*. J. Schmidt (ed.). Berkley, CA, University of California Press.

Francis, R. (2013a). *Report of the Mid Staffordshire NHS Foundation Trust Public Inquiry: Executive Summary*. London, House of Commons. HC 947.

Francis, R. (2013b). *Report of the Mid Staffordshire NHS Foundation Trust Public Inquiry: Volume III Present and Future Annexes*. London, House of Commons. HC 898-III.

Freud, S. ([1920] 1984). Beyond the pleasure principle. *On Metaspychology: The Theory of Psychoanalysis*. Harmondsworth, UK, Penguin Freud Library Series. Vol. 11.

Freudenberger, H. J. (1974). " Staff burn-out." *Journal of Social Issues* 30(1): 159–85.

Friborg, O., O. Hjemdal, Rosenvinge Jan H. and M. Martinussen (2003). "A new rating scale for adult resilience: what are the central protective resources behind healthy adjustment?" *International Journal of Methods in Psychiatric Research* 12(2): 65–76.

Gaffney, R. (1982). Letter from Florence Nightingale to Sir Thomas Watson, Bart, London dated 19 Jan 1867 in *Women as Doctors and Nurses. Health Care as Social History, Aberdeen* p. 139. O. Checkland and M. Lamb (eds). Aberdeen, UK, Aberdeen University Press: 134–48.

Gill, N. (8 January 2016). "Student nurses prepare to march as anti-fees campaign swells." *Guardian Students* Retrieved 6 July 2016, from www.theguardian.com/education/2016/jan/08/student-nurses-march-nhs-bursary-campaign

Gillespie, B. M., W. Chaboyer, M. Wallis and P. Grimbeek (2007). "Resilience in the operating room: Developing and testing of a resilience model." *Journal of Advanced Nursing* 59(4): 427–38.

Gillespie, B. M., W. Chaboyer and M. Wallis (2009). "The influence of personal characteristics on the resilience of operating room nurses: a predictor study." *International Journal of Nursing Studies* 46(7): 968–76.

Goffman, E. (1959). *The Presentation of Self in Everyday Life.* Harmondsworth, UK, Penguin.

Grandey, A. A. (2003). "When 'the show must go on': Surface acting and deep acting as determinants of emotional exhaustion and peer-rated service delivery." *Academy of Management Journal* 46: 86–96.

Greenwood, J. (1993). "The apparent desensitisation of student nurses during their professional socialisation: a cognitive perspective." *Journal of Advanced Nursing* 18: 1471–79.

Griffiths, P., J. Ball, T. Murrells, S. Jones and A. M. Rafferty (2016). "Registered nurse, healthcare support worker, medical staffing levels and mortality in English hospital trusts: A cross-sectional study." *British Medical Journal Open* 6:e008751 doi:10.1136/bmjopen-2015-008751.

Gullestad, S. E. (2001). "Attachment theory and psychoanalysis: Controversial issues." *The Scandinavian Psychoanalytic Review* 24: 3–16.

Gutteridege, N. (2016). "Calais migrants using makeshift RAFTS to cross channel as Britain braces for fresh influx." Retrieved 12 July 2016, 2016, from www.express.co.uk/news/uk/655706/Calais-migrants-refugees-Jungle-makeshift-rafts-cross-channel-Britain-UK-immigration

Habermas, J. (1984). *Theory of Communicative Action.* London, Heinemann Education.

Hagell, E. (1989). "Nursing knowledge: women's knowledge. A socio-logical perspective." *Journal of Advanced Nursing* 14(3): 226–33.

Hallam, J. (2000). *Nursing the Image.* London, Routledge.

Health Education England (2014). *Evaluation of Values Based Recruitment (VBR) in the NHS: Literature Review and Evaluation Criteria.* London, NHS HEE.

Helper, L. (2015, 19 October 2015). "Van Jones on the green jobs gap and what's wrong with resilience." Retrieved 1 November 2015, from www.greenbiz.com/article/van-jones-green-jobs-gap-and-whats-wrong-resilience

Hendrich, A., M. P. Chow, B. A. Skierczynski and Z. Lu (2008). "A 36-hospital time and motion study: How do medical-surgical nurses spend their time?" *The Permanente Journal* **12**(3): 25–34.

Hochschild, A. (1983). *The Managed Heart*. Berkeley, CA, University of California Press.

Hodges, H. F., A. C. Keeley and P. J. Troyan (2008). "Professional resilience in baccalaureate-prepared acute care nurses: first steps." *Nursing Education Perspectives* **29**(2): 80-89.

Hoel, H. and C. L. Cooper (2000). Destructive conflict and bullying at work. Unpublished report. Manchester, UK, Manchester School of Management UMIST.

Horkheimer, M. (1972). "Traditional and critical theory." *Critical Theory: Selected Essays*. New York, Seabury Press: 188–243.

Howell, A. and J. Voronka (2012). "Introduction: The Politics of Resilience and Recovery in Mental Health Care." *Studies in Social Justice* **6**(1): 1–7.

Ipsos MORI. (2016, 22 January 2016). "Politicians are still trusted less than estate agents, journalists and bankers: Ipsos MORI Veracity Index 2015: Trust in professions." Retrieved 6 July 2016, from www.ipsos-mori.com/researchpublications/researcharchive/3685/Politicians-are-still-trusted-less-than-estate-agents-journalists-and-bankers.aspx - gallery[m]/1/

Jacelon, C. S. (1997). "The trait and process of resilience." *Journal of Advanced Nursing* **25**(1): 123-129.

Jackson, D., A. Fau-Firtko and M. Edenborough (2007). "Personal resilience as a strategy for surviving and thriving in the face of workplace adversity: a literature review." *Journal of Advanced Nursing* **60**(1): 1–9.

James, N. (1989). "Emotional labour: skill and work in the social regulation of feelings." *The Sociological Review* **37**(1): 15–42.

Jamison, L. (2014, 26 August 2014). "Against Empathy." *Forum*. Retrieved 16 January 2016, from http://bostonreview.net/forum/against-empathy/leslie-jamison-response-against-empathy-leslie-jamison

Jennings, B. M. (2008). "Work stress and burnout among nurses: Role of the work environment and working conditions." *Patient Safety and Quality: An Evidence-Based Handbook for Nurses*. R. G. Hughes (ed.). Rockville MD, Agency for Healthcare Research and Quality (US): 134–48.

JM Consulting Ltd. (1998). *The Regulation of Nurses, Midwives and Health Visitors; Report on a Review of the Nurses, Midwives & Health Visitors Act 1997*. Bristol UK, JM Consulting.

Johnson, J. L. and S. A. Wiechelt (2004). "Introduction to the special issue on resilience." *Substance Use and Misuse* 39(5): 657–70.

Jones, C. B. (2005). The costs of nurse turnover: Part 2. Application of the nursing turnover cost calculation methodology. *Journal of Nursing Administration* 35(1), 41–9.

Karasek, R., C. Brisson, N. Kawakami, I. Houtman, P. Bongers and B. Amick (1998). "The Job Content Questionnaire (JCQ): An instrument for internationally comparative assessments of psychosocial job characteristics." *Journal of Occupational Health Psychology* 4(4): 322–55.

Kavanagh, D. (2006). "Pressure groups and policy networks." *British Politics*. D. Kavanagh, D. Richards, A. Geddes and M. Smith (eds). Oxford, Oxford University Press: 417–40.

Keogh, B. (2013). *Review into the Quality of Care and Treatment Provided by 14 Hospital Trusts in England: Overview Report*. London, NHS: 61.

Koen, M.P., C. van Eeden and M.P. Wissing (2011). "The prevalence of resilience in a group of professional nurses." *Health SA Gesondheid* 16(1): 1–11.

Larrabee, J. H., Y. Wu, C. A. Persily, P. S. Simoni, P. A. Johnston, T. L. Marcischak, C. L. Mott and S. D. Gladden (2010). "Influence of stress resiliency on RN job satisfaction and intent to stay." *Western Journal of Nursing Research* 32(1): 81–102.

Latour, B. (1987). *Science in Action: How to Follow Scientists and Engineers through Society*. Cambridge, MA, Harvard University Press.

Leveson The Right Honourable Lord Justice (2012). *An Inquiry into the Culture, Practices and Ethics of the Press: Executive Summary and Recommendations* [Leveson report]. London, The Stationery Office.

Levine, L. (1863). *International Commercial Law : Being the Principles of Mercantile Law of the Following and Other Countries, viz.: England, Scotland, Ireland, British India, British Colonies, Austria, Belgium, Brazil, Buenos Ayres, Denmark, France, Germany, Greece, Hans Towns, Italy, Netherlands, Norway, Portugal, Prussia, Russia, Spain, Sweden, Switzerland, United States, Wurtemburg*. London, V. and R. Stevens, Sons, and Haynes.

Lindsey, R. A. (2013). "What the Arab Spring tells us about the future of social media in revolutionary movements." Retrieved 23 November 2014, from http://smallwarsjournal.com/jrnl/art/what-the-arab-spring-tells-us-about-the-future-of-social-media-in-revolutionary-movements

Lintern, S. (2013). "HEE bids to tackle staffing crisis." Retrieved 25 August 2015, from www.hsj.co.uk/news/exclusive-hee-bids-to-tackle-staffing-crisis/5065750.article?blocktitle=News&contentID=13251-.Uph0U6NFAdU

Lintern, S. (2015). "Shock as NICE halts work on nurse staffing levels guidance." *Nurse Managers*. Retrieved 24 July 2016, from www.nursingtimes.net/roles/nurse-managers/shock-as-nice-halts-work-on-nurse-staffing-levels-guidance/5085546.fullarticle

Luthar, S. S. and D. Cicchetti (2000). "The construct of resilience: Implications for interventions and social policies." *Development and Psychopathology* 12(4): 857–85.

McDonald, G., D. Jackson, L. Wilkes and M. H. Vickers (2012). "A work-based educational intervention to support the development of personal resilience in nurses and midwives." *Nurse Education Today* 32(4): 378–84.

McDonald, G., D. Jackson, L. Wilkes and M. H. Vickers (2013). "Personal resilience in nurses and midwives: Effects of a work-based educational intervention." *Contemporary Nurse* 45(1): 134–43.

McDonald, L. (2005). *Florence Nightingale on Women, Medicine, Midwifery and Prostitution*. Waterloo, ON, Wilfrid Laurier University Press.

McGann, S. (1992). *The Battle of the nurses: A study of eight women who influenced the development of professional nursing 1880–1930*. London, Scutari Press.

Maben, J., S. Latter and J. M. Clark (2007). "The sustainability of ideals, values and the nursing mandate: Evidence from a longitudinal qualitative study." *Nursing Inquiry* 14(2): 99–113.

Mackintosh, C. (2006). "Caring: The socialisation of pre-registration student nurses: A longitudinal qualitative descriptive study." *International Journal of Nursing Studies* 43(8): 953–62.

Mance, H. (3 June 2016). "Britain has had enough of experts, says Gove." *Politics & Policy* Retrieved 24 July 2016, www.ft.com/content/3be49734-29cb-11e6-83e4-abc22d5d108c

Manzano García, G. and J. C. Ayala Calvo (2012). "Emotional exhaustion of nursing staff: Influence of emotional annoyance and resilience." *International Nursing Review* 59(1): 101–107.

Marmot, M. (2010). *Fair Society, Healthy Lives: The Marmot Review. Strategic Review of Health Inequalities in England post-2010*. London, University College London (UCL): 242.

Marx, K. (1845). "Thesis on Feuerbach." Retrieved 31 August 2015, from www.marxists.org/archive/marx/works/1845/theses/

Marx, K. and F. Engels ([1888] 1984). *The Communist Manifesto*. Harmondsworth, UK, Penguin Books.

Maslach, C., S. E. Jackson and M. P. Leiter (1996). *MBI: The Maslach Burnout Inventory: Manual*. Palo Alto, CA, Consulting Psychologists Press.

Masten, A. S. (2007). "Resilience in developing systems: Progress and promise as the fourth wave rises." *Development and Psychopathology* 19(3): 921–30.

Masten, A. S. and J. Obradovic (2006). "Competence and resilience in development." *Annals of the New York Academy of Sciences* 1094(1): 13–27.

Matos, P. S., L. A. Neushotz, M. T. Q. Griffin and J. J. Fitzpatrick (2010). "An exploratory study of resilience and job satisfaction among psychiatric nurses working in inpatient units." *International Journal of Mental Health Nursing* 19(5): 307–12.

Matthews, J. (23 November 2010). "Hospital patients 'left to drink water from vases'." Retrieved 12 July 2016, from www.express.co.uk/news/uk/213177/Hospital-patients-left-to-drink-water-from-vases

Maxwell, C., L. Brigham, J. Logan and A. Smith (2011). "Challenges facing newly qualified community nurses: A qualitative study." *British Journal of Community Nursing* 16(9): 428–30, 432–24.

Mealer, M., J. Jones, J. Newman, K. K. McFann, B. Rothbaum and M. Moss (2012). "The presence of resilience is associated with a healthier psychological profile in intensive care unit (ICU) nurses: Results of a national survey." *International Journal of Nursing Studies* 49(3): 292–99.

Media Reform Coalition (2014). Media Ownership Reform – A case for action, A Report on Media Ownership in the UK and the Case for Pluralism (produced jointly by MRC, NUJ, TUC and CPBF in November 2014). Retrieved 8 July 2016, from www.mediareform.org.uk/resources/media-ownership-reports

Meleis, A. (1985). *Theoretical Nursing: Development and Progress*. Philadelphia, PA, J B Lippincott.

Melia, K. M. (1987). *Learning and Working: The Occupational Socialization of Nurses*. London, Tavistock.

Menzies, I. E. P. (1960). "A case study in the functioning of social systems as a defence against anxiety: A report on a study of the nursing service of a general hospital." *Human Relations* 13: 95–121.

Mercer, S. W. and W. J. Reynolds (2002). "Empathy and quality of care." *British Journal of General Practice – Quality Supplement* 52: S9–S13.

Milmo, C. (2015). "Margaret Thatcher feared sex references in 1980s HIV campaign harmed nation's moral well-being: Archive documents reveal cabinet rows over public education programme." *UK Politics* Retrieved 24 July 2016, from www.independent.co.uk/news/uk/politics/margaret-thatcher-feared-sex-references-in-1980s-hiv-campaign-harmed-nations-moral-well-being-a6789946.html

Molina, Y., J. C. Yi, J. Martinez-Gutierrez, K. W. Reding, J. P. Yi-Frazier and A. R. Rosenberg (2014). "Resilience among patients across the cancer continuum: Diverse perspectives." *Clinical Journal of Oncology Nursing* 18(1): 93–101.

Moriarty, A. and P. Toussieng (1976). *Adolescent Coping.* New York, Grune & Stratton.

Morse, J. M., G. Anderson, J. L. Bottorff, O. Yonge, B. O'Brien, S. M. Solberg and K. H. McIlveen (1992). "Exploring empathy: A conceptual fit for nursing practice?" *Image: The Journal of Nursing Scholarship* 24(4): 273–80.

Murphy, L. and A. Moriarty (1976). *Vulnerability, Coping and Growth: From Infancy to Adolescence.* New Haven, CT, Yale University Press.

National Nursing Research Unit (2010). "Interruptions to nurses during medication administration: Are there implications for the quality of patient care?" *Policy*, Issue 22, London, King's College London.

Navarro, V. (2007). "Neoliberalism as a class ideology; or, the political causes of the growth of inequalities." *International Journal of Health Services* 37(1): 47–62

Nelson, S. (1995). "Humanism in nursing: The emergence of the light." *Nursing Inquiry* 2(1): 36–43.

Nelson, S. and S. Gordon, eds. (2006). *Complexities of Care: Nursing Reconsidered. The Culture and Politics of Health Work.* New York, Cornell University Press.

Neocleous, M. (2013). "Resisting resilience." *Radical Philosophy* 178: 2–7.

Commissioning Board Chief Nursing Officer and DH Chief Nursing Adviser (2012). *Compassion in Practice: Nursing, Midwifery and Care Staff, Our Vision and Strategy.* Leeds, Department of Health.

Nutting, M. and L. Dock (1907). *A History of Nursing: The Evolution of Nursing Systems from the Earliest Times to the Foundation of the First English and American Training Schools.* London, G. P. Putnam's Sons.

O'Malley, P. (2009). "Responsibilization." *The Sage Dictionary of Policing.* A. Wakefield and J. Fleming (eds). London, Sage: 276–77.

Olsen, D. P. (1991). "Empathy as an ethical and philosophical basis for nursing." *Advances in Nursing Science* 14(1): 62–75.

Paley, J. (2002). "Caring as a Slave Morality." *Journal of Advanced Nursing* 40(1): 25–35.

Paley, J. (2014). "Cognition and the compassion deficit: The social psychology of helping behaviour in nursing." *Nursing Philosophy* 40(4): 274–87.

Paley, J. (2015). "Francis, fatalism and the fundamental attribution error: A reply to Philip Darbyshire." *Nurse Education Today* 35(3): 468–73.

Paterson, J. and L. Zderad (1976). *Humanistic Nursing*. New York, John Wiley.

Porritt, L. (1990). *Interaction Strategies: An Introduction for Health Professionals*. Harlow, UK, Longman.

Prime Minister's Commission (2010). *Front Line Care: Report by the Prime Minister's Commission on the Future of Nursing and Midwifery in England*. London, Department of Health.

Rafferty, A. M. (1993). "Decorous didactics: early explorations in the art and science of caring c. 1860-90." *Nursing: Art and Science*. A. Kitson (ed.). London, Chapman and Hall: 48–84.

Rafferty, A. M. (1996). *The Politics of Nursing Knowledge*. London, Routledge.

Reeves, J. (2002). *Writing Alone, Writing together: A Guide for Writers and Writing Groups*. Novato, CA, New World Library.

Rius (1994). *Marx for Beginners*. Cambridge, Icon Books.

Rogers, C. R. (1959). A theory of therapy, personality, and inter-personal relationships as developed in the client-centered framework. Reprinted in 1989. *The Carl Rogers Reader*. H. Kirschenbaum and V. Henderson (eds). Boston, MA, Houghton Mifflin.

Rutter, M. (1985). "Resilience in the face of adversity: Protective factors and resistence to psychiatric disorder." *British Journal of Psychiatry* 147: 598–611.

Schaufeli, W. B., M. P. Leiter and C. Maslach (2008). "Burnout: 35 years of research and practice." *Career Development International* 14(3): 204–20.

Sermeus, W., L. H. Aiken, K. Van den Heede, A. M. Rafferty, P. Griffiths, M. T. Moreno-Casbas, R. Busse, R. Lindqvist, A. P. Scott, L. Bruyneel, T. Brzostek, J. Kinnunen, M. Schubert, L. Schoonhoven, D. Zikos and R. C. Consortium (2011). "Nurse forecasting in Europe (RN4CAST): Rationale, design and methodology." *BMC Nursing* 10: 6.

Simms, A. (18 April 2016). Junior doctors contract: Jeremy Hunt's legal power to impose new contract questioned. *The Guardian*. London.

Smith, A. (1904). *An Inquiry into the Nature and Causes of the Wealth of Nations*. London, Methuen.

Smith, P. (1992). *The Emotional Labour of Nursing*. Basingstoke, UK, Macmillan Education.

Snow, S. and E. Jones. (8 March 2011). "Immigration and the National Health Service: putting history to the forefront." *Policy Papers* Retrieved 1 August 2016, from www.historyandpolicy.org/policy-papers/papers/immigration-and-the-national-health-service-putting-history-to-the-forefront

Stockholm Resilience Centre (2012). *What is Resilience? An Introduction to Social-Ecological Research*. Stockholm, Sweden, Stockholm Resilience Centre.

Stone, J. (27 November 2015). "George Osborne actually cut public health budget by 20 per cent despite NHS promises, analysis finds." *UK Politics*. Retrieved 3 August 2016, from www.independent.co.uk/news/uk/politics/george-osborne-actually-cut-health-budget-by-20-per-cent-despite-nhs-promises-analysis-finds-a6751311.html

Stone, J. (18 March 2016). "Budget includes £650 million in 'secret cuts' to the NHS, analysis shows." *UK Politics*. Retrieved 3 August 2016, from www.independent.co.uk/news/uk/politics/nhs-cuts-budget-george-osborne-secret-stealth-privatisation-a6938441.html

Strong, P. and J. Robinson (1990). *The NHS – Under New Management*. Milton Keynes, UK, Open University Press.

Traynor, M. and A. Evans (2014). "Slavery and jouissance: Analysing complaints of suffering in UK and Australian nurses' talk about their work." *Nursing Philosophy* 15(3): 192–200.

Traynor, M., K. Stone, H. Cooke, J. Maben and D. Gould (2013). "Disciplinary processes and the management of poor performance among UK nurses: Bad apple or system failure? A scoping study." *Nursing Inquiry* 21(1): 51–8.

Tusaie, K. and J. Dyer (2004). "Resilience: A historical review of the construct." *Holistic Nursing Practice* 18: 3–10.

Van Dijck, J. (2013). *The Culture of Connectivity: A Critical History of Social Media*. Oxford, Oxford University Press.

Verhaeghe, P. (1999). *Love in a Time of Loneliness: Three Essays on Drive and Desire*. London, Karnac Books.

Wagnild, G. and H. M. Young (1990). "Resilience among older women." Image: *Journal of Nursing Scholarship* 22(4): 252–55.

Waldman, D., F. Kelly, S. Arora and H. Smith (2004). "The shocking cost of turnover in healthcare." *Health Care Management Review* 35(3): 206–11

Weber-Newth, I. and J.-D. Steinert (2006). *German Migrants in Post-War Britain: An Enemy Embrace*. Oxford, Routledge.

Westbrook, J .I., C. Duffield, L. Li and N. J. Creswick (2011). "How much time do nurses have for patients? A longitudinal study quantifying hospital nurses' patterns of task time distribution and interactions with health professionals." *BMC Health Services Research* **11**(1): 1–12.

Wheeler, B. (16 January 2014). "Whatever happened to the happiness agenda?" Retrieved 31 October 2015, from www.bbc.co.uk/news/uk-politics-25746811

Willis, P. (2012). Quality with Compassion: *The Future of Nursing Education. Report of the Willis Commission on Nursing Education.* London, Royal College of Nursing: 55.

Willis, P. (2015). *Raising the Bar, Shape of Caring: A Review of the Future Education and Training of Registered Nurses and Care Assistants*, Leeds, Health Education England.

Winders, S. (2014). "From extraordinary invulnerability to ordinary magic: A literature review of resilience." *Journal of European Psychology Students* **5**(1): 3–9.

Witz, A. (1990). "Patriarchy and professions: The gendered politics of occupational closure." *Sociology* **24**: 675–90.

Woolgar, S. (1988). *Science: The Very Idea.* Chichester, UK, Ellis Horwood.

Zander, M., A. Hutton and L. King (2010). "Coping and resilience factors in pediatric oncology nurses." *Journal of Pediatric Oncology Nursing* **27**(2): 94–108.

Zimbardo, P. (2007). *The Lucifer Effect: How Good People Turn Evil.* London, Rider.

Žižek, S. (2005). "Beyond discourse analysis." *Interrogating the Real.* London, Continuum: 271–84.

Index